LYME DISEASE ALTERNATIVE TREATMENTS

Natural Remedies, Holistic, Herbal Approaches for Chronic Lyme

Herb Roi Richards

Taylore Vance

Terms and Conditions

Table of Contents

Introduction

Lyme disease is a complicated disease that is often initially misdiagnosed as many different diseases until a proper diagnosis is arrived at; only then will the patient have any understanding that they have a chronic life-long condition for which there is no cure.

Many stories abound about the origin of the disease, which is no concern to the students of this course material. The fact is, Lyme Disease is here. The American Medical Association's stand on the matter is that there is no known cure for the disease, and the best we can do is pharmacologically treat the symptoms in patients as they arise; this is the medically approved treatment for Lyme Disease.

This course aims to introduce the greater medical community to options for treating Lyme disease outside the boundaries of traditional medical treatment modalities based on data and testimonials obtained from our Lyme disease conferences and personal experiences.

Medical doctors and practitioners who have personally suffered from the burden of having Lyme disease have sought help outside their prescribed dictates to manage their conditions, and most of them have found alternative healing methods to address their concerns and the varying disorders associated with the disease.

Even if a medical professional has benefitted from these alternative medicines or therapies, they are not likely to refer them to their patients for fear of potentially losing their ability to practice medicine, which is their livelihood.

And so it goes, not only for those working in the medical arts but also for the normal citizenry of the United States of America, who are also discouraged from claiming they have benefitted greatly from these alternatives to authorized medical interventions.

People who have Lyme disease can suffer significantly from the disease and are likely to look to everything from which doctor to see – to consider visiting a witch doctor – and everything in between.

The overwhelming testimonial evidence shows that these natural remedies and alternative medicines can effectively treat and possibly eliminate Lyme disease.

The jury is still out because neither the government nor the American Medical Association will spend American dollars to come to a logical conclusion. Instead, the government considers most, if not all, of the alternatives you will learn about in this course as unorthodox, potentially dangerous to the bottom line of the pharmaceutical companies they've chosen to invest in.

This information is provided to the medical community as information only.

You may receive continuing education credit for attending these classes but may choose not to claim it, and we understand your situation.

If you are a practicing medical professional, you are advised not to discuss what you learn about alternative treatments for Lyme disease here. You may seek someone outside your practice to refer your patients to for alternative therapy for conditions associated with Lyme disease.

Healing Practitioner credentials are offered along with this course to religiously protect non-medical professionals from harassment by the government for speaking about the medical alternatives mentioned in the course. Thanks to the separation of church and state, medical licensure may still be at risk for medical professionals who also possess the Healing Practitioner credential.

By continuing to access the rest of the course material, you understand and agree that we are not providing you with any medical advice whatsoever. This information is intended for medical professionals only to raise their awareness about non-medical treatments and therapies that are neither sanctioned by the American Medical Association nor any governing faction of the United States government.

If you suffer from Lyme disease, seek a natural healthcare professional for advice.

Chapter 1:

Symptoms and Misdiagnosis of Lyme Disease

We have agreed to skip over the source(s) of Lyme disease and the conditions that may spread the disease to its current status as being an incurable disease growing among the population of America and the world, with the Center for Disease Control or CDC, reporting 30,000 new cases of Lyme disease every year.

Most agree that the number of medical cases of Lyme disease in the United States is grossly understated, as Western Europe reports 230,000 patients suffering from Lyme disease. As a medical professional, you may already know that 30,000 is incorrect because your current client base does not align with these statistics.

A minimum of 300,000 Lyme disease patients would be a more accurate number for the United States, and this number is growing at a rate of over 800 per day, which makes it a contender as being a toxic and chronic disease that cannot simply be confined to being "passed by deer ticks" as the propaganda suggests.

Regardless of its origins, or how it has epidemically spread so rapidly around the world, and the fact that there reportedly is "no known cure," when it becomes chronic, people from all walks of life, even medical professionals who may be suffering from Lyme disease are seeking alternative methods to battle this medical anomaly that shows up with the symptoms of most every disease known to man.

Symptoms of Lyme disease span an entire spectrum of conditions, often accompanied by extreme pain and suffering. The symptoms can be masked by prescribed pharmaceutical solutions, only to have another completely different symptom occur shortly after that; this is a continual cycle of treatment in a rinse-and-repeat fashion, which can have the patient drowning in little brown bottles in no time.

Symptoms of Lyme Disease

There are so many symptoms of Lyme disease that it's no wonder patients are misdiagnosed with other diseases. For example, here is a list of the top 50 symptoms of Lyme disease.

Top 50 Symptoms of Lyme Disease

- ☐ Abdominal pain or poor digestion
- ☐ Arthritis-type conditions
- ☐ Bladders, irritable or poor function
- ☐ Blurry vision, sensitive to light
- ☐ Brain fog
- ☐ Breast pain, unexplained milk production
- ☐ Concentration difficult
- ☐ Cramps or pain in muscles
- ☐ Ear pain, sensitive to sounds
- ☐ Exaggerated symptoms, i.e., "worst ever..." for certain conditions

- ☐ Eye inflammation
- ☐ Flu-like symptoms
- ☐ Forgetfulness
- ☐ Getting lost, hard to find car in parking lot
- ☐ Headache
- ☐ Hear/feel cracking when turning neck
- ☐ Heart problems, such as an irregular heartbeat
- ☐ Joint & back stiffness
- ☐ Knee or hip replacement
- ☐ Lethargy
- ☐ Liver inflammation
- ☐ Loss of appetite
- ☐ Mood swings, anger, depression
- ☐ More sensitive to alcoholic drinks
- ☐ Muscles twitching: especially in face
- ☐ Nausea
- ☐ Neck pain or stiffness
- ☐ Occasional vertigo, poor balance
- ☐ Pain or swelling in joints: Which ones?
- ☐ Pelvic Pain or testicular pain
- ☐ Pulse skips
- ☐ Regularity changes – diarrhea, constipation
- ☐ Sexual – loss of libido, dysfunction

- ☐ Short term memory poor
- ☐ Skin rash
- ☐ Sleep disturbances – Sleep apnea, wake early etc.
- ☐ Sore ribs or pain in chest
- ☐ Sore throat
- ☐ Sudden need to lie down or sit
- ☐ Suddenly unable to spell simple words
- ☐ Swollen glands
- ☐ Swollen lymph nodes
- ☐ Swollen tissue, rashes, oozing fluid
- ☐ Tingling in hands, feet, or back
- ☐ Tiredness, lack of stamina, fatigue
- ☐ Tremors
- ☐ Unusual chills, fevers, sweats or flushing
- ☐ Unusual hair loss
- ☐ Unusual menstrual irregularity for ladies
- ☐ Unusual weight loss or gain

The most common symptoms are arthritic challenges. One-third of all patients with Lyme disease will initially report physical symptoms such as stiffness and joint pain, physical sensitivity or tenderness at areas around the joints, reduced mobility, development of bone spurs, or a feeling as though joints are not moving as smoothly as before as if they have lost lubrication or are "getting rusty."

Other arthritic complaints include swelling around joint areas, pain in joints of hands, wrists, and feet, often mirrored on both sides of the body, and joint inflammation.

The range and severity of Lyme disease's symptoms vary widely from patient to patient, almost as if each case were an individual work of art, where no two are the same.

Factors that seem to affect the level of suffering in the Lyme disease patient seem to be complicated by other factors and sensitivities that the patient might possess, such as a compromised immune system, other bacterial infections, poor cellular protection and function, and exposure to environmental conditions that could make symptoms worse.

Exposure to parasites, mold, or toxins would create complications and increase the severity of Lyme disease symptoms.

All these factors make an accurate early diagnosis of Lyme disease nearly impossible.

Misdiagnosis of Lyme Disease

With so many symptoms, who would blame you for misdiagnosing anyone with Lyme disease? Your patient comes in with clear and exact indications of suffering from a particular disease. You prescribe the proper medication to treat the symptoms of the disease, and it responds appropriately; this is a win for any physician.

It is widespread for a patient with Lyme disease to say, "I was first misdiagnosed with," followed by any of the common misdiagnoses for what eventually becomes discovered to be Lyme disease. The first is likely followed by other diagnoses for new symptoms as they arise. But to be fair, these are not misdiagnosing at all.

For all intents and purposes, these are proper diagnoses, and Lyme disease does respond to the prescribed treatment. However, it doesn't end there. Lyme disease finds another place to fester and creates another set of symptoms that can be treated appropriately and probably respond also.

Misdiagnosis is understandable and expected and is not a sign of quackery, as some sufferers of Lyme Disease might conclude. The medical community comprises professionals trained to investigate the available data, reasonably conclude a diagnosis based on a hypothesis, and establish a treatment regimen to help ease the patient's condition.

The professionally trained medical community is competent in this area. Based on the information provided by the patient and the results of any testing, the doctor comes to a conclusion and treats the condition based on the information. There is no lack of competency in doing so.

As a normal course of action, a competent treating physician would follow the same process if the patient developed new symptoms.

Unless the medical professional is aware that Lyme Disease might be the culprit, he or she may continue to diagnose and treat the symptoms as they appear.

Most people seem to believe that when the spirochete that causes what is now called Lyme disease learned to piggyback in ticks and other biting insects, it forgot how to transfer from host-to-host by close personal contact, just like it has done for centuries. Granted, this is a slightly different spirochete from the one that causes syphilis and the one causing relapsing fever, but they are still spirochetes.

That could explain how so many people have Lyme disease who have never been in the forest or been bitten.

Now, you know, if a patient's file is full of a laundry list of different diagnoses in succession, chronic Lyme disease is a potential proper diagnosis.

Chapter 2:

Medical Response to Lyme Disease

The medical technologies available for diagnosing Lyme disease are still in their infancy and must be more accurate. Reportedly, combinations of the Western blot and ELISA tests can help diagnose Lyme disease in some patients by measuring specific antibodies; this appears to work on some patients but not all, so accurate diagnosis is still essentially a part of the attending physician's investigative research.

By far, the best sign of Lyme disease for early diagnosis is the appearance of a bullseye rash surrounding the area of a bite from an infected tick, though twenty percent of patients do not develop the bullseye rash. Hundreds of victims of Lyme disease have never been bitten by anything, so there is no reason for suspicion that they may have it.

Once you have a diagnosis of Lyme disease, there is a medical response that practitioners follow when treating someone with the disease.

The attending physician will prescribe an antibiotic regimen for the patient.

According to the Centers for Disease Control (CDC), most patients who have contracted Lyme disease from a tick will positively respond to antibiotics, such as a combination of amoxicillin, cefuroxime axetil, or doxycycline, taken over a course of two to four weeks.

The best results of an antibiotic regimen will be seen by those who are treated immediately following infection. Admittedly, this is not an effective protocol for all patients, as in more than half of the people who contract the disease, it can lay dormant for some time, not being expressed symptomatically, while spreading stealthily throughout the central nervous system.

The longer it spreads without symptomatic expression, the less effective antibiotics will be, and the patient is none the wiser because they have no idea anything is wrong during this secret gestation period.

For those who respond to early antibiotic therapy, recovery is often rapid and complete.

Early detection and intervention are the key to success in treating Lyme disease. Although, there are some complications that can occur even with early detection and antibiotic treatment. For instance,

Some people are antibiotic-resistant or allergic to antibiotics. Antibiotics may cause side effects or may not be able to be used in some patients who may be pregnant.

Long-term use of antibiotics may do more harm than good. As they kill harmful and good bacteria necessary for an effective immune system, they may promote the unchecked growth and spread of Lyme disease throughout the central nervous system.

For the other patients, who will chronically suffer a variety of symptoms over time, they are diagnosed with post-treatment Lyme disease (PTLD), and the road to treatment and recovery can be tedious, long, and painfully traveled.

According to the Centers for Disease Control (CDC), prevention is the best hope for controlling Lyme disease. Not contracting it is the most effective method of controlling it; to prevent getting Lyme disease, the CDC suggested that you,

Use Bug Repellant

Using a bug repellant when you are out in nature will keep mosquitos at bay and the deer tick, which is known to transmit the disease to humans, at bay. These repellants should also be used while working in the garden, enjoying the beach, hiking in the woods, or camping.

Wear Tick-safe Attire

You should wear clothing that covers most of your skin, such as long-sleeved shirts, long pants, tall socks, and white or light-colored clothing. This way, you can easily spot a tick and rid yourself of it before it reaches a vulnerable location to bite you.

Check Yourself

If you've been out in open areas with a tick population, be sure to check yourself when you get back inside for ticks. If you find them, remove them immediately.

Pregnant?

Pregnant women should avoid any areas populated with ticks due to potential complications in treating Lyme disease in patients with children.

No Known Approved Cure for Chronic Lyme Disease

Unfortunately, there is no known approved cure for Lyme disease. Therefore, patients and the medical community are often found outside the boundaries of traditional medical advice, looking for answers in nature or elsewhere for relief. Many who've done just that have proven that relief is available.

Chapter 3:

Natural Treatment of Chronic Lyme Disease

Patients, and even their doctors, who have chronic Lyme disease (CLD) or post-treatment Lyme disease (PTLD) may become highly frustrated with the treat-the-symptom approach to managing the condition for which there is no known cure.

There are some natural approaches to self-care that can reduce the symptoms of the ongoing chronic conditions associated with those suffering the long-term effects of Lyme disease.

Treating Lyme Disease Naturally

1. Diet and Exercise

Eating a healthy diet can help build your body's natural ability to fight off disease and significantly reduce Lyme disease symptoms. Exercise is also known to create a super immune system. Combining the two can put you on the path to managing the long-term effects of Lyme disease and may even lead to a healthy recovery.

Stop Eating Inflammatory Food

Certain foods propagate inflammation, such as sugar, fruit, and grains.

- ☐ Sugar
- ☐ Fruit
- ☐ Grains

By restricting your diet to exclude these foods known to promote adverse effects on the same target areas that are breeding grounds for Lyme disease, you are taking a proactive approach to limit the spread and impact of an otherwise rampant spread of Lyme disease.

Start Eating Non-Inflammatory Food

Just as there are foods that promote inflammation, there are also foods that are anti-inflammatory and essentially put the fire out. These foods can help you combat the effects of inflammation, which is often a key component of Lyme disease's attack on its human host.

Among these foods are,

- ☐ Vegetables
- ☐ Nuts
- ☐ Seeds
- ☐ Organic meat
- ☐ Coconut
- ☐ Raw cultured dairy
- ☐ Bone broth

You should add more vegetables, nuts, seeds, organic meat, coconut, raw cultured dairy, and bone broth to your diet and avoid foods that cause inflammation, pummeling the Lyme disease dragon at every meal.

Immunity-building Food

If you want a highly-empowered immune response to anything Lyme disease has to throw your way, then eating foods known to boost your immune system is key.

It is well-known that foods high in their anti-oxidant capabilities are a practical approach to supporting a super-powered immune system. Start building your immunity by eating more,

- [ ] Vegetables
- [ ] Fresh (locally sourced) fruit
- [ ] Berries
- [ ] Dark leafy greens
- [ ] Brightly-colored vegetables

These are just a few of the foods that are known to boost your immune system.

Probiotics

When you take antibiotics, you may be attacking both harmful and beneficial bacteria. These good bacteria are known as probiotics, and certain foods can replenish the bacteria necessary to battle Lyme disease.

Most yogurt has good probiotic content; the more organic, the better. Yogurt made from goat's milk appears to have the highest content of probiotics.

Other probiotic foods include kefir, amasai (fermented unpasteurized cow's milk), and fermented vegetables such as kimchi, sauerkraut, and kvass.

2. Supplements

Your body needs the basic raw materials to combat the effect of Lyme disease, especially for long-term sufferers, so daily supplementation is critical to see that you have the nutrients that provide the tools necessary to do the work.

Vitamin D3

If you're battling Lyme disease, you should spend some time in the sun to boost your Vitamin D. If you can't get out in natural sunlight, you can supplement by taking Vitamin D3 orally, about 5,000 IU.

B Vitamins

B-complex vitamins significantly increase cellular function and metabolic supremacy, enabling you to increase your neurological abilities and fight infection. Vitamin B-6 is at the top of the list for reducing stress and fatigue for people with Lyme disease.

Potassium & Magnesium

Potassium and magnesium are essential for maintaining proper electrolyte levels for a healthy heart. Patients with Lyme disease are often deficient in magnesium and potassium, so don't let them be counted among them. Supplement with a good over-the-counter product.

Omega-3s

Omega-3 fatty acids are the rock stars of chronic Lyme disease patients by boosting brain function, including cognitive ability and overall neurology. You'll achieve this by eating foods like nuts, seeds, and wild-caught fish, for example, or doing over-the-counter omega-3 supplementation.

CoQ10

CoQ10 is another neurological booster that protects the brain from inflammatory attacks of Lyme disease and reduces inflammation in the lower extremities.

About 200 mg twice a day is the recommended daily portion for sufferers of Lyme disease, fibromyalgia, and other autoimmune diseases.

3. Take a Nap

You must preserve your natural resources, so pay attention to getting your zees every night. Start finding ways to get better sleep at night, and don't be embarrassed at all about taking a nap during the day. Some of the world's best, most powerful people take a mid-day nap. You'll be surprised how much more natural energy you will have just by taking a 20-minute power nap during the day.

4. Don't Worry, Be Happy

Reduce Stress

Stress feeds the Lyme disease beast, so pay attention to areas in your life that might be stressful, and take time to restructure your life to reduce the stressors in your life. Eliminate worry and emotional stress from your life, both triggers for Lyme attacks.

Have Fun

As a natural approach to battling chronic Lyme disease, having fun reduces stress and creates opportunities to have even more fun. Lyme disease hates joy because when you are really happy, your immune system gets a substantial hormonal jolt, which knocks Lyme disease for a loop.

Being really, really happy could be the key to overcoming your otherwise lifetime struggle with Lyme disease.

5. Environmental Control

Find ways to put yourself in the driver's seat of your life. If there are environmental areas of your life that are putting you at risk, you need to take charge and protect yourself from things that could make your Lyme disease struggle any harder than it already is.

Bug-a-boos

Parasites, viruses, bacteria, and other infectious pathogens are known to empower Lyme disease to make you suffer unbearably and ruin your life by adding its negative power to anything that would cause a problem for anyone without Lyme disease; this makes you more susceptible to exaggerated responses which are many times more painful than anyone without the disease.

Structure your life to avoid exposure to parasites, viruses, bacteria, and other infectious pathogens.

Mold

Mold is the mother of yuck. If you don't reduce your mold exposure, you will inadvertently feed the Lyme disease monster. Plus, mold is just bad. Mold can cause nasal congestion, throat or eye irritation, coughing, wheezing, or, in some cases, skin irritation in otherwise healthy individuals.

Some people are more sensitive to mold than others, but if you have chronic Lyme disease, you will be particularly sensitive to the effects of mold and will experience more severe reactions to it.

Chapter 4:

Introduction to Alternative Treatment

The First Steps in Alternative Treatment

In this segment, we will introduce you to the first phase of alternative treatment modalities that have been effective in treating chronic Lyme disease (CLD) or post-treatment Lyme disease (PTLD).

These methodologies are thought to be of little or no risk, and the consensus of the standard medical community may view them as ineffective. The results obtained from them are more likely related to the Placebo Effect.

Holistic health practitioners are more likely to offer some of the following remedies to their treatment regimens for Lyme disease. They are also expected to use a direct microscopy test from Fry Labs in Arizona (frylabs.com). It is inexpensive and more accurate when combined with other physical testing than other tests commercially available to the standard medical community.

Other nutritional supplements offer additional relief and benefits to those with long-term Lyme disease.

Natural Diet

While the previous segment mentioned diet and healthy eating, this time, you want to take the idea of eating healthy to another level; this includes eating only natural, locally sourced foods, less cooking that depletes the nutrients of the food, avoiding charring of food, and using microwaves in the cooking process.

Avoid sugar and pre-packaged foods, and avoid drive-through restaurants. Consume convenience or fast foods while integrating more healthy fats into your diet.

Different people benefit from other approaches to eating healthy, so experimentation is necessary to find out what works best for you.

Probiotics

In addition to consuming foods containing natural probiotics infuses the body with more probiotics over the counter or in other forms is highly effective in treating Lyme disease.

Consuming 50 billion units of probiotics, including at least eight different strains, appears to noticeably decrease the severity of Lyme disease symptoms.

Turmeric

Turmeric is a spice as well as a medicinal herb, serving as a natural anti-inflammatory that greatly decreases the pain associated with painful joints, headaches, damaged blood vessels, and nerves.

Mushrooms

Medicinal mushrooms, such as cordyceps, reishi, and maitake mushrooms, are added to the anti-Lyme disease regimen, as they are known for boosting the immune system, reducing inflammation and stress due to their ability to enhance a particular intracellular antioxidant known as SOD (superoxide dismutase) which protects the cells from attack.

This variety of mushrooms also empowers the natural human cells that attack and kill bad bacteria to do so more efficiently.

Ashwagandha

Adding an ashwagandha supplement to the Lyme disease regimen is warranted because it is an effective herbal method of naturally reducing stress and balancing cortisol levels throughout the body.

Parasite-killing Herbs

There is a group of herbs that are particularly good at killing off parasites known to complicate or worsen the effects of Lyme disease. Some of those commonly suggested are,

- ☐ Black walnut
- ☐ Garlic
- ☐ Grapefruit seed extract
- ☐ Oregano
- ☐ Wormwood

Other natural treatment regimens that target parasites and the infections that accompany them include,

Activated Charcoal

Activated charcoal (carbon) is believed to have properties that treat parasites, a wide range of toxins, and other harmful substances that may create problems for both those who suffer from Lyme disease and those who do not.

Bentonite Clay

Like activated charcoal, Bentonite clay is often suggested for its ability to bind with chemicals and heavy metals, allowing them to be eliminated through the digestive system without lingering and festering inside the body.

Symptomatic Herbal Therapy

Different herbs have different effects on the body. The patient can express difficulty in one area or experience pain or other challenges in other parts of the body, even having trouble managing cognitive resources.

Whatever the patient's complaint, there is likely an herbal remedy that will help to relieve pain or discomfort with any challenge the patient may face. Symptomatic herbal therapy is not the be-all and end-all in the treatment of Lyme disease, but it can lessen the discomfort of Lyme disease enough to encourage the patient to continue the process of getting better and bolster hope of one day being free of Lyme disease altogether.

Essential Oils

The use of essential oils to deploy and administer healing herbs, flowers, and other plants is growing in the holistic healing community. It is coming into its own in the new culture of modern folk medicine.

Essential oils and other aroma therapy methods are becoming increasingly common in most American households.

Practice Forgiveness

Picking up where the last segment left off on not worrying and stress reduction, the practice of forgiveness can go a long way toward health and healing. There is no better way to reduce worry, bad feelings, or stress than forgiving others.

Keep in mind that forgiving others does not require an apology or blessing. Forgiveness happens within you and yourself, and it is not intended for those who need forgiveness or punishment, as God better issues these.

Your forgiving others is for you, a private matter between you and your heart. Also, remember to find forgiveness for yourself in all things, as unforgiveness for one's self or guilt are potent stressors that trigger Lyme disease.

Even More Stress Reduction

Other methods of reducing or eliminating stress include meditative practices, joining a support group, journaling, taking a walk, initiating and maintaining a regular exercise program, and finding time to relax in natural settings outdoors.

- ☐ Meditate
- ☐ Join a group
- ☐ Journal
- ☐ Take a walk
- ☐ Exercise
- ☐ Relax in nature

Again, everyone is different, as is exemplified by the fact that everyone's case of Lyme disease is unique. That is why determining what works best for each person requires extensive trial and error, but it is worth it.

Chapter 5:

Rejected Alternative Treatment and Therapies

The next phase of alternative treatments and therapeutic modalities is so innovative that the Centers for Disease Control, the Food and Drug Administration, and the National Institutes of Health have taken a proactive stance to reject the idea of using any of these treatments to battle the effects of Lyme disease entirely.

Basically, the anti-Lyme-disease-alternative-therapies trifecta (CDC, FDA, and NIH) have categorized these rejected methodologies into five categories: (1) Oxygen, (2) Energy and Radiation, (3) Heavy Metals and Chelation, (4) Nutritional and Herbal, and (5) Biological and Miscellany.

The general stance of these government agencies represents the idea that there is no empirical scientific research data to confirm that any of these alternative treatments for Lyme disease are effective in any way. The people who promote them are predatory and seek to defraud and profit from the ill who are sick and dying, preying on their weakened condition, offering little more than false hope. Not unlike snake oil salespeople back in the day.

In some cases, the FDA has banned some of these Lyme disease treatment alternatives and, in other cases, made them illegal to promote or use at all.

The Cure for Lyme Disease

Let it be known that we are not making any claims that there is a known cure for Lyme disease. The most curious thing about these rejected alternative treatments for Lyme disease is that for those American citizens who have dared to use them, a surprising and growing number are expressing, "I found the cure for Lyme disease!"

Their testimonials are nearly miraculous, and they claim that some of these rejected methodologies even eliminate Lyme disease completely.

Of course, suppose you suffered with battling the Lyme disease monster for many years without relief and suddenly found relief, possibly never to have the monster knock on your door ever again. In that case, you might feel like shouting your experience from the rooftops in an effort to share your discovery with others.

Immediately, if not sooner, the claims of these individuals are silenced by various methods.

Attack the Patient

Others viciously attack the individuals who seek to share their stories, some health care professionals, and other people who are vehemently opposed to using any alternative therapies. Those who have experienced positive results are ridiculed and bullied for even considering alternative treatment, and if they have shared their experience via social media, they risk its deletion, claiming some "violation of user agreement."

We understand that this person's story is purely anecdotal and that they understandably may possess some excitement about achieving some relief from the ongoing struggles and pain associated with long-term Lyme disease.

Any of us might feel enthusiastic about sharing the things in our lives that make us feel good or triumphant, but we rarely are attacked, ridiculed, or bullied for doing so.

Attacking the patient is an excellent method of silencing the individual who has experienced positive results from an alternative Lyme disease treatment.

Most sufferers of Lyme disease over time are not loud-mouthed proponents of anything. They have struggled with pain and suffering for a long time. Many people cannot understand why they should be suffering for so long, and they are used to dealing with a certain degree of disapproval from friends, family, and healthcare professionals.

There is a certain degree of post-traumatic stress disorder that accompanies any long-term illness, so any patient thereof may be easily intimidated, even easily frightened, to speak their truth, whatever it may be.

Throw in a couple of keywords, like,

Idiot - Illegal - Dangerous - Fatal

And the patient may run and hide, never to utter another word about their recovery.

A job well done for the opponents of alternative therapies, which leaves believers wondering who is really behind all this violent negativity. It's no wonder that a number of these people rush to the idea that conspiracy may be underlying such outbursts.

It is not the intent of this course to claim or uncover the existence of any conspiracy, only to note that it is understandable that someone who has received positive results from trying an alternative treatment for Lyme disease might not be openly forthcoming about their results.

Nonetheless, many of these alternative therapies do seem to have varying degrees of success among those who have used them to combat the long-term suffering from Lyme disease.

We will introduce you to some of the methodologies the Centers for Disease Control, the Food and Drug Administration, and the National Institutes of Health rejected.

1, Oxygen

     a)   Hyperbaric oxygen chambers
     b)   Ozone therapies
     c)   Hydrogen peroxide

2, Energy and Radiation

     a)   "Photon" therapy
     b)   Magnet therapy
     c)   "Rife" therapy

3, Heavy Metals and Chelation

     a)   Chemical chelation
     b)   Silver
     c)   Bismuth

4, Nutritional and Herbal

     a)   Vitamins and herbs

b) Magnesium and serrapeptase

c) Marijuana and cannabis oil

5, Biological and Miscellany

a) Urine therapy

b) Enema therapy

c) Sodium chlorite solution

Chapter 6:

Rejected Lyme Disease Treatments

This segment will examine the Top 15 rejected Lyme disease alternative treatments.

Note that the following methodologies are not sanctioned by the Centers for Disease Control (CDC), the Food and Drug Administration (FDA), or the National Institutes for Health (NIH) for treating Lyme disease or any other disease within the borders of the United States of America.

The Top 15 Rejected Lyme Disease Treatments (In no particular order)

- Hyperbaric oxygen chambers
- Ozone therapies
- Hydrogen peroxide
- "Photon" therapy
- Magnet therapy

- "Rife" therapy
- Chemical chelation
- Silver
- Bismuth
- Vitamins and herbs
- Magnesium and serrapeptase
- Marijuana and cannabis oil
- Urine therapy
- Enema therapy
- Sodium chlorite solution

Let's take a closer look at these banned alternative treatments.

1. Hyperbaric oxygen chambers

A hyperbaric oxygen chamber can vary in size from a one-person tube to an entire room that can house many people. The area housing the patient(s) is pressurized as it is filled with medical-grade oxygen. This methodology is used to get more oxygen to the tissues for those who suffer from decompression sickness, burns, diabetic wounds, carbon monoxide poisoning, and some other types of infections.

Lyme disease patients do report positive results from Hyperbaric Oxygen Therapy (HBOT) and claim that the process kills anaerobic bacteria by increasing oxygen while improving immune function and repairing damaged tissues.

Treatment times vary anywhere from 45 minutes to 2 hours once a week, every two weeks, or once a month, based on the patient's needs. Each treatment will cost $100 or more per visit and may or may not be covered by insurance (depending on your coverage and its restrictions).

2. Ozone therapies

Ozone therapy may be recommended for patients with Lyme disease. It reportedly has a noticeable positive effect on those particularly suffering from joint pain, fatigue, and brain fog while boosting the immune system. This methodology employs the use of ozone (O3 instead of regular oxygen, which is O2). The intent is to deliver more oxygen to the cells of the body through the ozone therapy process.

When ozone is administered intravenously, the patient's blood is extracted, mixed with ozone, and replaced by an intravenous drip. Ozone (O3) may also be administered orally, rectally (as a gas), directly onto the skin (as gas, in water, or an oil-base), or via a hyperbaric chamber, and is often used in conjunction with other naturopathic therapies.

Ozone therapy can be taken bi-weekly at a cost of $75 to $250 or more per treatment, depending on the method of administration.

3. Hydrogen peroxide

Hydrogen peroxide intravenous infusion is heralded by those affected with Lyme disease as a relief from persistent symptoms. Other methods of getting hydrogen peroxide into your system include oral ingestion and transdermal applications, though IV infusion has the best results.

Patients report positive results from hydrogen peroxide (H2O2) in reducing inflammation, joint pain, fatigue, brain fog, and relief from sleep deprivation.

An infusion takes 1 to 2 hours and can start with weekly infusions, tapering off to bi-weekly, monthly, or bi-monthly, depending on how well the Lyme disease patient progresses. Each treatment will cost $100 or more per visit.

4. Photon therapy

The basis of photon therapy relies on a type of electromagnetic light (biophotons) that quantum sciences uncovered as having therapeutic value based on its interconnectivity with all life. This spectrum of infrared light is the method by which all cells communicate with one another.

This is the basis of the Bionic 880 photon therapy machine used to deploy the biophotons to patients with Borreliosis (Lyme disease), which reduces the body's biophotons overall. Restoration of the body's biophotons repairs damaged cells and is facilitated by bi-weekly photon therapy treatments. Noticeable improvements are reported after three to five treatments.

A photon therapy session lasts 90 minutes to two hours and costs about $100 per session. Alternatively, you can get your own Bionic 880 for about $13,000.00.

5. Magnet Therapy

Magnet therapy for Lyme disease varies widely. On one end of the spectrum, you have magnetic bracelets and other forms of magnetic jewelry; on the other, you have magnetic mats or beds upon which the patient lies while treatment sessions are performed. In between is the intuitive system (using kinesiology) of applying magnets of varying sizes and strengths to specific body part locations singly or in pairs.

There are a variety of certification and non-board-approved licenses for specifically branded magnetic therapeutic modalities for treating diseases, some targeted to chronic diseases, like long-term Lyme disease.

Sessions initially range from 90 minutes to two hours, but they are reduced to 45 minutes to an hour for regular maintenance. Depending on the provider, expect to pay about $100 per session or more.

6. Rife Machine

Users of the Rife machine report therapeutic results for various diseases, including Lyme disease. Inventor Royal Raymond Rife developed this electronic frequency generator nearly a hundred years ago, which applies different electronic signals to the patient to foster healing.

Compared with newer alternative healing modalities, there is a huge number of anecdotal testimonials collected over the course of a century of use as a treatment intervention for patients who are less responsive to traditional medicine.

This frequency treatment identifies the electronic frequency of the patient's complaint and counteracts it by applying electromagnetic energy to the affected area, which theoretically cancels out the malady or kills off the threatening cells.

A wide variety of Rife machines are available, costing thousands of dollars, and treatment sessions run in the $60.00 per hour range.

7. Mercury Toxicity Therapy

Mercury toxicity therapy or chelation therapy operates from the assumption there exists a connection between toxic levels of mercury in the body, which complicate and prolong diseases, including Lyme disease, and making them reach long-term and chronic stages, which would not be suffered by those without some form of mercury poisoning.

Holistic practitioners (and some medical professionals) believe that removing toxic mercury from the body by various methods, including removing amalgam dental fillings, will return the patient to harmonic balance and rid them of chronic disease.

The process begins with an evaluation by a holistic practitioner or other proactive licensed or unlicensed practitioner who then recommends a treatment program that likely includes the removal of silver fillings and a detoxification regimen. This regimen may consist of chemical chelators for eliminating heavy metals and varies widely depending on the practitioner.

8. Colloidal Silver

For over 1,200 years, colloidal silver, also known as silver water, which has tiny silver particles in it, has been used as a bactericide. There was a resurgence in the use of colloidal silver among the medical community as it was being used in hospitals as an antibacterial agent in the 1900s, and this continued until patented antibiotics replaced silver took its place between the 1930s and 1940s.

Since then, it has remained popular as a staple of folk medicine and among holistic practitioners. Many Lyme disease patients claim a noticeable reduction in symptoms of chronic Lyme disease (CLD) or post-treatment Lyme disease (PTLD) by consuming colloidal silver as a regular supplement to their normal health maintenance program.

The highly germicidal silver water is non-toxic and generally safe for human consumption. A one-month supply is in the neighborhood of thirty to fifty dollars.

9. Bismuth

Despite the evidence that ranitidine bismuth citrate (RBC) is effective in killing B. burgdorferi in the cyst and motile forms, the FDA has deemed it dangerous and potentially causes death in patients with Lyme disease. Meanwhile, long-term sufferers of Lyme disease praise the results and benefits of using Bismuth in the treatment of their chronic symptoms.

It might be prohibited from being used in the United States. Still, injectable versions of Bismuth, such as bismacine, chromacine, Bismacine-C, and Bismacine-N, are available for treating Lyme disease outside the USA, even though it may cause bismuth poisoning, leading to kidney or heart failure.

Bismuth is available over-the-counter and taken orally, as well as Pepto-Bismol (bismuth subsalicylate), bismuth subnitrate, bismuth subgallate, and others. These offer some benefits, but the best testimonials regarding Bismuth administered by injection are reported.

10. Vitamins, Minerals, and Herbs

Holistic, naturopathic, and nutritional practitioners often recommend large amounts of vitamin C and B-12 for treating Lyme disease, followed by B6, folate (B9), D3, A, and E vitamins, minerals magnesium (Mg) and chromium, coenzyme Q10, and omega-3 fatty acid supplements.

Herbal recommendations for those struggling with Lyme disease include curcumin, Rhodiola rosea, cat's claw, cinnamon bark, chlorella, clove bud, oregano, garlic, olive leaf, teasel root, cilantro, and sarsaparilla.

While using vitamins, minerals, and herbal supplements to treat disease may seem counter-intuitive for mainstream medical practitioners, for those stacking supplements to mitigate the damages of their suffering from Lyme disease, there is little or no risk of harming themselves. For the people who use them, their results are more than satisfying.

11. Enzyme Therapy

How do enzymes help those with Lyme disease? Lyme seeks to hide behind a protective biofilm, which makes it invisible to any supplement you might be taking, thus preventing your efforts to render it impotent or cause Borrelia burgdorferi's death. Enzymes penetrate the biofilm, removing the cloak of invisibility so your proactive approach to battle Lyme can perform accordingly. Lumbrokinase is an enzyme derived from earthworms that reportedly does impact those with Lyme disease. Twenty milligrams (mg) of lumbrokinase twice daily does the trick. Another enzyme therapy that is highly beneficial in the battle against Lyme disease is nattokinase, an enzyme derived from soybeans. The nattokinase dosage is higher than lumbrokinase, like 250 mg daily. Serratiopeptidase (AKA serrapeptase) is in 30 mg dosages and is commonly taken in conjunction with nattokinase, taken twice a day, 30 mg serrapeptase with 125 mg of nattokinase.

Check with your natural doctor first, especially if you are taking a blood thinner regimen, as this is a known contraindicator.

12. Marijuana and Cannabis Oil

Marijuana contains THC, which can be helpful in making the painful symptoms of chronic Lyme disease more manageable. The potential downside of using marijuana is that THC can also get you high, which could cause impairment, and you should not drive, operate heavy equipment, enter into an agreement, or sign your name on any document if you are "stoned." Other warnings about using marijuana include not taking marijuana if the patient has been diagnosed with a mental disorder because marijuana can cause psychosis or worsen an ongoing mental disorder.

Cannabis oil, also known as cannabidiol or CBD, has no, or very low, levels of THC and is currently legal in all 50 states of the USA; this seems to be an acceptable method of achieving the medicinal results obtained by using marijuana without the high.

Because both marijuana and cannabis oil lower blood pressure, those who have heart disease or currently have low blood pressure should not take marijuana or CBD oil as they may increase the risk of heart attack.

13. Urine Therapy

As you may have guessed, urine therapy centers around drinking one's urine. While the thought of drinking your urine would understandably make anyone squeamish, there is a growing group of people who believe in drinking their own, and some claim to enhance their spirituality by engaging in this practice.

Many people have prolonged Lyme disease who swear by it. Some studies confirm the efficacy of a urine therapy protocol for many diseases besides Lyme disease, and anecdotal evidence abounds.

14. Enema Therapy

Of all the types of enemas, the coffee enema ranks at the top among Lyme disease patients inclined to use them. Enemas are an excellent way to remove toxins from the body, especially those in the liver, and the colon cleanse is generally accepted as a valid detoxification method.

Chronic Lyme disease patients report the immediate effects offer a great deal of relief, though most report the effects do not last long, so they might go through three or more rounds of coffee enemas per day to achieve the desired results.

Proceed with caution. Those who have had negative experiences with coffee enemas complain of coffee being too hot, rectal tears, and infections. These can be avoided by using room-temperature coffee, lubricating the enema wand with castor or coconut oil, using purified water, and sanitizing equipment following use.

15. Miracle Mineral Solution (MMS)

Miracle Mineral Solution, or MMS, as it is commonly referred to, is a Chlorine Dioxide Solution (ClO_2). Many treatment-resistant Lyme disease patients claim prolonged use of this inexpensive product, commercially available over-the-counter as a water purifier treatment, and report being no longer plagued by Lyme disease.

The FDA is vehemently opposed to the use of MMS or CDS by Americans to treat any disease, such as Lyme disease, claiming it is industrial bleach that could burn or cause seriously harmful side effects, including the possibility of killing anyone who ingests it.

While the FDA refuses to honor the use of MMS or
CDS to treat any disease, it is authorized for use as an
antimicrobial agent (that's why it's a common
ingredient in toothpaste and mouthwash). The
Centers for Disease Control (CDC) encourages adding
it to public water to make it safe to drink. It is
approved for use worldwide by the Environmental
Protection Agency (EPA) as a water purifier. It is
recommended for use by the World Health
Organization (WHO) for drinking water treatment.
The Food and Drug Administration (FDA) has
approved it for use to ensure safety in food
preparations and drug formulations.

For those who claim to no longer have any signs of
ongoing Lyme disease symptoms who have used
MMS or CDS, it's no wonder they are confused about
the mixed signals.

Chapter 7:

Energy Healing Modalities for Lyme Disease

This segment will examine the Top 15 energy healing modalities Lyme disease patients use. These patients report success in obtaining relief from symptoms of chronic Lyme disease, and some claim to no longer have Lyme disease at all thanks to these esoteric, energetic approaches to healing.

Note the following methodologies are not sanctioned by the Centers for Disease Control (CDC), the Food and Drug Administration (FDA), nor the National Institutes for Health (NIH) for treating Lyme disease or any other disease within the borders of the United States of America. Even so, open-minded hospitals invite energy healing practitioners, like Reiki Masters, to come and administer healing to patients. Of the reasons for doing so, more rapid patient recovery times and "feeling better" during the patient's hospital stay are atop the list.

The Top Energy Healing Modalities for Lyme Disease

1. Acupressure
2. Acupuncture
3. Chakra Healing
4. Cranio-sacral Therapy
5. EFT, or Emotional Freedom Techniques®
6. Healing Touch (HT)
7. Lomi lomi
8. Polarity Therapy
9. Pranic Healing
10. Quantum Touch®
11. Reiki
12. Laser Reiki
13. Restorative Touch™
14. Shamanic Healing
15. Shiatsu

Take a closer look at these energy-healing modalities for treating Lyme disease.

1. Acupressure

How does acupressure help the body?

Acupressure is a health procedure used in China thousands of years ago as traditional Chinese medicine. Evidence shows that it was even older and practiced in the Stone Age!

It's a method of activating the body's self-healing mechanisms to treat illness and alleviate pain. Like acupuncture, which uses tiny needles, acupressure is applied pressure that stimulates the body at certain meridians or pressure points.

What is Acupressure? – WebMD Says:

Acupressure has been used for over 2,000 years in China. It applies the same principles as acupuncture to promote relaxation and wellness and to treat disease. Sometimes called pressure acupuncture, acupressure is often thought of as simply acupuncture without the needles.

Acupressure is conducted by applying finger pressure anywhere without special equipment.

You can treat yourself with very little practice. Acupressure should be applied slowly and gently. Using it too quickly or vigorously can create discomfort, especially in the abdominal area.

Acupressure strengthens the immune system and promotes wellness.

Acupressure also reduces nausea in cancer patients receiving chemotherapy.

Correctly performed, acupressure increases circulation, reduces tension and pain, and relaxes the body.

Special care and caution are needed in the case of a pregnant woman or in treating a person with burns, infections, and recent injuries.

Acupressure is more effective than physical therapy for most patients with low back pain.

Ear acupressure can be used to reduce stress and anxiety.

Acupressure is used to reduce fear and anxiety in trauma victims and pre-operative care.

Acupressure can be beneficial to treat all these conditions:

- Decreased Libido
- Migraine Headaches
- Tension Headaches
- Toothache
- Jaw Pain
- Earache
- Neck Pain
- Shoulder Pain
- Wrist Pain
- Hand Pain
- Arm Pain
- Hip Pain
- Knee Pain
- Ankle Pain
- Foot Pain
- Backache
- Constipation
- Diarrhea
- Heartburn

- Stomachache
- Loss of Voice
- Colds
- Flu
- Sore throat
- Sinus Infection
- Bed-wetting
- Incontinence
- Urinary retention
- Allergies
- Depression
- Anxiety Attacks
- Nervousness
- Hiccoughs
- Insomnia
- Hangover
- Fainting
- Reduce nausea and vomiting in children
- Improve memory and concentration
- High blood pressure
- Angina
- Heart palpitations
- Hot flashes
- Pregnancy discomfort

- PMS
- Painful periods
- Morning sickness
- Nose bleeding
- Itching
- Asthma

Here are a couple of acupressure tips you can try:

For a painful knee joint, put a tennis ball on a pillow, then place your leg over it, pushing it into the crease behind your knee. Find the sensitive spot just below your kneecap and slightly to the outside of the shinbone. Press into it gently with your fingertips for about one minute.

For headaches and muscle or joint pain, press the fleshy part of your hand between your thumb and index finger. Hold this for one minute, then repeat on the other hand.

For low-back pain, lie on your back with your feet propped up on a sofa or chair. Place two tennis balls under your lower back on either side of your spine. (I got cheap tennis balls in the dog toy department.)

Stay in this position for about one minute.

How to Massage Your Pressure Points

When you have a painful spot, what do you do?
You reach for it.

Without conscious thought, your hand often goes to the discomfort area and massages it. Your hands have energy vortexes that give out healing streams of energy. (This flow can be amplified. See Reiki.)

Learning the simple basics of acupressure could make this mindless self-massage even more beneficial. It can help you relax and manage chronic pain.

"The Chinese medical model discovered that these invisible lines of energy crisscross the human body."

"This theory also holds that each meridian pathway connects to each of your organs. This interconnection of specific points allows acupressure to alleviate pain and promote healing."

In nine of ten studies, many have found acupressure effective at reducing pain.

With an ancient track record, this method of pain management has undoubtedly stood the test of time.

Getting Started

When using acupressure to apply self-massage, you must be consistent and patient. Improvements may not be immediate, but regular acupressure massage can reduce pain and the likelihood of recurrences.

When using acupressure:

Sit or lie down in a comfortable position.
Relax, close your eyes, and breathe deeply.
Set aside several minutes.
Use firm, deep pressure in a slight rotating or up-and-down movement.

Do You Have Lower Back Pain?

Two main pressure points can help with lower back pain.

The first is on your waist:

Stand up and lightly grab your waist with both hands so your thumbs wrap around your back.

With your thumbs in place, apply a circular motion with thumbs using firm pressure for a count of five seconds.

Repeat this three times.

You can also find a pressure point to relieve low back pain about midway up your calf muscle:

Using the same circular motion and pressure, hold for five seconds.

Release and repeat two more times.

For Achy Shoulder Pain

Neck and shoulder pain are often the result of stress and can lead to migraines and tension headaches. Several pressure points, beginning with one of the most commonly used positions, can relieve shoulder pain.

"The first and easiest to find is between the web of the

thumb and the first finger."

Press with firm pressure until you feel a mild ache.

Hold for five seconds.

Release and repeat three more times.

For those with Sinus Pain

The first point for relieving sinus pressure and pain is right between your eyebrows, says Moreau. He suggests using your index finger or thumb to apply pressure here using a circular motion for 5 seconds.

The second point is at your temples; use the same circular motion as before.

A third option is to trace your fingers from your temples to either side of your nostrils. Using a circular motion, apply pressure here for five seconds.

Moreau recommends following this pressure technique for each pressure point, keeping the pressure firm but not painful.

Final Tips on Acupressure

These practices are done several times each day, but it is wise to give your body a break if any points are sore to the touch. It would be best to start with light pressure and gradually move to a firmer touch.

Tension and stress often cause feelings of pain. Relaxing and reducing stressors is essential for these approaches to have the most impact. If you find relaxing and simultaneous self-massage challenging, you can always ask for help from a friend or family member.

You can learn to do acupressure at home to supplement professional treatment. This procedure is especially useful when you are stricken with illness or pain and cannot get to the doctor when you need help.

2. Acupuncture

How does acupuncture work?

ANSWER: Acupuncture improves the body's functions and energy flow. It promotes natural self-healing by stimulating the body's specific anatomic sites and pressure points. The most common method to stimulate "acupoints" is the insertion of fine, sterile needles as thin as a single hair into the skin.

Were there Stone Needles?

Today, acupuncture needles are made from stainless steel and are usually thrown away after every use. But did you know that these needles were initially made of wood sticks, bamboo, bones, and even stone? Yes, it's true!

While the thought of shaping stones can be perplexing, ancient acupuncturists used stone needles during acupuncture. The only catch is that these stone needles were less thin than modern ones.

Healing Power of Acupuncture

Acupuncture helps align your energy. It is an ancient form of Chinese medicine that uses different pressure points of your body. These pressure points provide various health benefits when activated, including helping muscle pain, allergies, chronic problems, and even increasing infertility.

Keep reading to learn more about acupuncture and how it can help you.

Why Would You Use Acupuncture?

You can benefit from getting acupuncture no matter what you have been experiencing lately, emotionally, mentally, or physically. Your whole body needs to work together. What often happens is that you treat one part of your body while another ache or pain is relieved simultaneously. The power of acupuncture is that it doesn't just treat one spot or muscle like your doctor does, it promotes healing and wellness throughout your whole body at once.

Top 10 Benefits of Acupuncture for Workplace Stress and Pain

- Reduced stress
- Reduced back pain and neck tension and relief of joint pain in the hands and arms
- Relief from headaches
- Reduced eye strain
- Improved immune system and reduced sick days
- Enhanced mental clarity and increased energy.
- Relief from digestive conditions
- Allergy relief

Your Tongue Says It All

During a visit to your doctor, they use equipment like a stethoscope and blood pressure monitor to help diagnose a person's health properly during checkups. Your acupuncturists will only have to look at your tongue to determine your present health condition.

They will also feel your pulse, as conventional doctors do, but they get all the information they need by looking at your tongue and devising the best treatment.

You can get relief from your

- Poor digestion
- Allergy symptoms
- Help with infertility issues
- It also is used for mood issues, stress, and depression.

How to Get an Acupuncture Treatment?

One of the biggest questions asked by people who have never seen it done is, "What exactly happens?" a valid question that can set your mind at ease.

When you hear that tiny needles are used, it can be scary, but this therapeutic practice, which has been practiced for centuries, is very healing and relaxing.

How quickly does acupuncture work?

In some cases, acupuncture needles are inserted and then removed a few seconds later. To feel the full benefits of the treatment, you will generally require approximately 6-12 acupuncture sessions. Most sessions last between 20 and 40 minutes.

When you go for an Acupuncture treatment, the practitioner first asks why you are getting it And What problems you are trying to alleviate.

There are different locations where acupuncture can be done for various aches or pains.

These needles are hair-thin, so you probably won't even feel them.

When your appointment comes, you will lie still and wholly relaxed on a massage table as each needle is placed at the proper pressure point. You will continue lying still to let the needles work their magic.

What You Should Know About Acupuncture?

You Might Need Several Sessions

Acupuncture usually works quickly for many people, but sometimes, treatments may be needed to achieve the full effects.

Do you take your clothes off for acupuncture?

You may not need to remove your clothes like you would for a massage to receive an Acupuncture treatment. However, they recommend wearing loose clothing so that sleeves can be rolled up above the elbows and pants legs can be pulled up above the knees.

You May Feel A Little Sensations

While it should not cause pain, sometimes, one needle might come too close to a nerve, causing a slight pain sensation.

Schedule Time Before and After Your Appointment

This treatment is relaxing and balancing. When you schedule your acupuncture appointment, be sure you have plenty of time and are not engaged in a stressful activity before or afterward. Besides, do not overbook yourself on the day of your appointment, as you want to relax during the acupuncture treatment.

Choosing The Right Acupuncturist

If you want to do research, if you feel wrong, don't

hesitate to choose someone else. Let your intuition be your guide.

Ask your friends on your health forum for suggestions. Choosing the right acupuncturist is like choosing any health professional.

Eat A Small Meal Amount Before Your Appointment

 You risk feeling lightheaded if you go to your appointment on an empty stomach, so eat something before your appointment. Most experts recommend eating a light meal approximately two hours before your treatment. Make sure this isn't too big a meal, as this may cause you to feel uncomfortable during your appointment.

How much does acupuncture cost?

Typical costs: An initial visit fee for an acupuncture session and medical consultation ranges from $75 to $95. Routine visits cost $50 to $70.

What are the side effects of acupuncture?

Out of millions who receive treatment annually, the

agency reports receiving only a few complaints per year about complications from acupuncture. As with any health treatment, acupuncture poses some risks. The most common situation is pain and bleeding from the insertion of acupuncture needles. Other adverse effects can include skin rashes, allergic reactions, bruising, nausea, dizziness, fainting, or infections.

What should you not do before acupuncture?

Avoid coffee Before Your Appointment.

Do not drink Caffeine for at least two hours before your Acupuncture treatment because it is a stimulant. Coffee increases your body's fight-or-flight response, which acupuncture seeks to lessen.

Does Insurance Cover Acupuncture?

More health insurance plans cover the Acupuncture treatment for chronic pain and other symptoms. Find out when it's covered. The alternative called acupuncture has come a long way since it was first introduced in the United States. Today, it's a natural alternative healthcare treatment often integrated with traditional medical care.

3. Chakra Healing

The Definition of Chakra

The word chakra means wheel or vortex. Chakras are seven energy centers in the body that control various energies and powers within. They are believed to spin like a flat plate from the front of the body to the back. The chakras control multiple aspects of body, mind, and spirit.

The Central Channel

The chakras are believed to be connected by the central channel, which allows energy to be moved up and down to aid in health and healing and help maintain overall balance.

The central channel is said to be located just in front of the spinal column and runs parallel to it, from the anus to the crown of the head.

The Subtle Energy Bodies

The chakras and central channels are part of what is termed the subtle energy body. If we were to perform surgery, we would not see the chakras or channels inside a person's body. They are not physical but help determine energy and overall health.

The Placement of the Chakras

There are 7 chakras, 3 lower and 4 higher. The three lower chakras deal with the body and are essentially our power base, making us physically strong and stable and helping us gain all our most essential needs. The 4 higher chakras have more to do with our mind and spirit.

The 7 chakras, with their location and energy, in order from bottom to top, are:

- Root - the anus, basic needs, such as food, warmth, and shelter.

Root Chakra- Red Color

Stability, Security, Grounding

If this chakra works optimally, you will feel

supported, connected, safe to the physical world, and grounded.

Emotional imbalances

Feeling worried about basic survival needs like money, work, food, and shelter.

There are physical symptoms of imbalance problems in the immune and digestion systems, legs, feet, prostate gland, rectum, male reproductive parts, and tailbone, among others.

> Sacral- the sex gland and reproductive organs, creativity

Sacral Chakra-Orange Color

Wave of Creativity, Pleasure, Spontaneous & Zest of Life, Feel Joy

You will feel committed, passionate, pleasurable, creative, abundant, and able to enjoy sex in your life if this chakra is optimally balanced.

Emotional imbalances

Ability to have sex and fun, express and control our emotions, and connect with people—fears of addictions, impotence, and betrayal.

Physical symptoms of imbalance

Sexual and reproductive issues, kidney dysfunctions, urinary problems, menstrual troubles, hip, pelvic, and lower back pain, and irritable bowel syndrome.

> Solar Plexus—the open area between the ribs on your midriff, representing your willpower, ability to get things done, and assertiveness.

Solar Plexus-Yellow Color

Will Power, Self-Control, Performer, Self-Acceptance

If this chakra is optimally balanced, you will feel optimistic, self-compassionate, assertive, calm, and confident.

Emotional imbalances

Issues of less willpower, self-worth, personal power, fear of physical appearance, criticism, and rejection.

Physical symptoms of imbalance

Colon diseases, liver and pancreas problems, digestive problems, chronic fatigue, liver dysfunction, diabetes, high blood pressure, stomach ulcers, gall stones, gluten intolerance.

> Heart - at the heart, your love and compassion

Heart Chakra-Green Color

Love & Relationship, Emotional Balance, Acceptance

If this chakra is optimally balanced, you will feel joy, compassion, love, gratitude, and peace.

Emotional imbalances

issues of heart, anger, jealousy, bitterness, suffocation, and fear of loneliness
Physical symptoms of imbalance

issues with breasts, heart problems, asthma, allergies, lymphatic systems, immune diseases, arm and wrist pain, upper back, and shoulder problems.

> Throat - at the throat, your ability to speak the truth, including your inner truth.

Throat Chakra-Sky Blue

Communication, Openness, Self Esteem

If this chakra is optimally balanced, you will feel truthful and honest yet firm, free to articulate your thoughts, feelings, and ideas.

Emotional imbalances

Inability to express or communicate about things that matter to you, inability to believe in your creativity.

Physical symptoms of imbalance

Thyroid issues, asthma, persistent sore throat, mouth ulcers, laryngitis, TMJ, throat infections, ear infections, or any facial problems, neck and shoulder pain.

> Third eye - at the space between the eyebrows, above the bridge of your nose. The third eye is the seat of your intuition and instinct.

Third Eye-Blue Color

Clarity in Thoughts, Intuition & Wisdom, Vision

When this chakra is balanced, we feel clear and focused, able to distinguish truth from illusion, and open to receiving wisdom and insight.

Emotional imbalances

Problems with self-reflection, moodiness and volatility, confusion, inability to think about other's points of view

Physical symptoms of imbalance

Blurred vision, headaches, sinus issues, hormone function, eyestrain, hearing loss, seizures, migraines.

> Crown - the top of your head, is your spiritual

connection with the universe.

Crown Chakra- Purple Color

Conscious Living, Awareness, Oneness, Ability to See Larger Picture

When this chakra is balanced, we live in the present moment and have unshakeable trust in our inner guidance.

Emotional imbalances

Problems with self-knowledge and power, anxiety, fear, depression and dissatisfaction, constant confusion

Physical symptoms of imbalance

Sensitivity to environment, light and sound, dizziness, and depression.

4. Cranio-sacral Therapy

What is Craniosacral therapy, and how does it work?

Craniosacral Therapy (CST) is a gentle, light touch, hands-on approach to assessing the craniosacral system. It involves gently touching various body locations to test for the ease of energy flow, motion, and rhythm of the cerebrospinal fluid pulsing around the brain and spinal cord.

That gentle touch releases tensions deep-seated in the body, improving whole-body health and performance. It relieves pain and dysfunction. Physician John E. Upledger, Osteopath, discovered and developed it after years of clinical testing for a wide range of medical problems that cause pain and symptoms of disease. He was a researcher at Michigan State University, where he served as a professor of biomechanics.

The trained CST practitioners use a soft touch, which is generally no greater than 5 grams - about the weight of a nickel - and practitioners use their hands to evaluate the craniosacral system. The practitioner gently feels various body locations to test for the cerebrospinal fluid's ease of motion and rhythm. The touch releases restrictions in the central nerve system by allowing the soft tissues to be felt. CST is a preventive health measure to bolster disease resistance for various medical complications associated with pain and dysfunction.

How Does a Craniosacral Treatment Work?

What is the central nerve system? The brain and spinal cord make up this system. The nerve system significantly influences the body's ability to function correctly. We must have free-flowing fluid throughout this nerve system. The craniosacral system heavily influences your health—the health of the membranes and fluid that surround, protect, and nourish the brain and spinal cord controls the system's efficiency.

Your body endures stresses and strains in everyday life, and it must work to compensate for them. Unfortunately, this tension and anxiety often cause body tissues to tighten and distort the craniosacral system. These distortions of stress can then cause pressure to form around the brain and spinal cord, resulting in restriction. This restriction can create a barrier to the healthful performance of the central nervous system and potentially with every other network where it interacts.

Help is as close as your CST clinic. Luckily, these stressful restrictions can be detected and corrected using simple methods of light touch. The CST practitioner uses a gentle touch to relieve restrictions in any tissues influencing the craniosacral system.

By normalizing energy flow and tissue, the environment around the brain and spinal cord can correct itself. CST enhances the body's ability to self-correct. Craniosacral Therapy can alleviate a wide variety of dysfunctions, from chronic pain and sports injuries to stroke and neurological impairment.

What conditions does Craniosacral Therapy address?

- Concussion and Traumatic Brain Injury
- Migraines and Headaches
- Chronic Neck and Back Pain
- Autism
- Motor-Coordination Impairments
- Stress and Tension-Related Disorders
- Chronic Fatigue

- Post-Traumatic Stress Disorder
- Infant and Childhood Disorders
- Brain and Spinal Cord Injuries
- ADD/ADHD
- Fibromyalgia
- TMJ Syndrome
- Scoliosis
- Central Nerve System Disorders
- Learning Disabilities
- Orthopedic Problems
- And Many Other Conditions where a flow of energy is needed

Is cranial adjustment safe?

Cranial adjustment and chiropractic care are very safe for both adults and children. Successful "adjustments" can significantly improve their quality of life. Children with cranial misalignment can suffer from speech and math problems, reading troubles, or even seizures and pain.

What is the craniosacral system?

The craniosacral system consists of the membranes and fluid surrounding and protecting the brain and spinal cord, as well as the attached bones. A trained specialist makes these adjustments. These important membranes extend from the bones of the skull, face, and mouth (which comprise the cranium) down the spine to the sacrum or tailbone area.

What is the cranial release technique?

A practitioner is available in your city to perform the Cranial Release Techniques (CRT). It is a natural, relaxed, gentle, hands-on approach to releasing the body's inborn capacity to heal and regenerate itself. The CRT works to restore proper function to the nerve system and proper balance to the body structure.

What do you wear to Craniosacral therapy?

You should wear loose-fitting, thin clothing. This way, the practitioner can better sense what's happening in your body. For the hands-on work to be most effective, you'll be asked to lie on your back on a massage table. The therapist evaluates your craniosacral rhythms by quietly resting your hands on your skull and sacrum.

Do you need a license to practice Craniosacral therapy?

Does the practitioner need to touch you? Yes. Most states require the practitioner to have a "license to touch a client" to practice craniosacral therapy, including licenses for massage therapy, physical therapy, occupational therapy, Reiki, etc.

How much does Craniosacral therapy cost?

A practitioner may offer a free consultation. Discount prepaid packages are available for clients who want to make Craniosacral Therapy a regular part of their health and wellbeing. After finding a practitioner, the fee for a one-hour session is $150, and an hour and a half is $225. (Appointments for children under 10 are typically 30 minutes and cost $75.)

5. EFT, or Emotional Freedom Techniques®

Emotional Freedom Technique

The Emotional Freedom Technique (EFT) is a tapping energy healing method based on the theory that our physical symptoms and emotions are linked to the underlying blocked energy system of the body. This system also uses the acupuncture meridian practice known to the Chinese for thousands of years.

Gary Craig, a Stanford Engineer, is the creator of EFT. Craig uncovered the underlying theory in 1991 and continues to build and improve EFT procedures today.

The underpinning theory of EFT is uncomplicated yet sheds a whole new light on our emotional experiences and how we interpret them. We stuff negative emotions in the physical body, where they become pain and disease.

Craig believes "our unresolved negative emotions are major donors to most physical pains and diseases." His EFT discovery statement asserts, "The cause of all negative emotions is a disruption in the body's energy system."

Use Your Fingertips

We like having you use both hands and all your fingers to tap. The fingers are gently relaxed and form a slightly curved natural line. Using more than two fingers allows you to access a larger area and more of the acupuncture points. It's better than just tapping with one or two fingertips. Using four fingers will allow you to cover the tapping points more quickly.

However, many obtain quite successful results with the traditional one-handed two-finger approach. You can use either method, but I tend to use my modified version to be complete.

Use your fingertips, not your finger pads, as they have more meridian points. However, you should use your finger pads if you have long fingernails.

How Does EFT Work to Relieve Pain?

The ancient Indian Science of Ayurveda and Chinese Medicine both support the concept that our emotional experiences contribute significantly to the development of disease in the human body.

Do you have resentments, hurts, and anger?

EFT is very easy to learn, and tapping will help you:

- Reduce Food Cravings
- Remove Negative Emotions
- Reduce or Eliminate Pain
- Implement Positive Goals

While the EFT approach that all negative emotions are caused by a disturbance in the body's energy system may sound unusual initially, the idea is far from new. It's over 5,000 years old and was more recently enforced by Albert Einstein, who taught that everything is made of energy.

Ramtha, an ancient being who cares about the human predicament, says everything is consciousness and energy!

EFT works well because it contains the secrets of Eastern healing traditions the West has overlooked.

Acupuncture and acupressure are finally attracting

attention, and modern research has been conducted to determine how and why it works. Here, all that research will seek to put Acupuncture and Acupressure in a box that makes sense to what conforms to Western logic. The results are so impressive that they have been referred to as a placebo effect by the uneducated when, in truth, they are the results of the ancient knowledge of meridian energy circuitry, which runs throughout all living creatures.

EFT - Linked to Acupuncture and Acupressure

In acupuncture, points are carefully selected by trained practitioners who understand the maps of the meridian system. The clearing practice of EFT tapping is based on a few of these strong points. These points give emotional and physical relief to anyone who learns where these simple points are and how to use them. This simple EFT doesn't require expert knowledge or the use of needles; the locations are stimulated by tapping on them with the fingertips.

For proof, we want only to look at the evidence that hundreds of people in China experience heart surgery utilizing only acupuncture for anesthesia. It is incredible to realize that anything based on a solid healing foundation, like acupuncture, has much to offer and is worth exploring.

Gary Craig developed EFT as an incredibly user-friendly access point to the benefits of acupuncture and the healing potential inherent within us all to deal with our physical and emotional pain. All you have to do is tap specific energy points on your face, side, and hands. EFT's track record for relieving pain, trauma, negative emotions, anxiety, and stress has earned it the original title of "acupuncture for the emotions, but without the needles."

The EFT Challenge Is to Help You Feel Better

When you try tapping with your fingertips, you are inputting kinetic energy onto specific meridians on the face, head, arms, and chest. At the same time, you verbalize and think about your particular problem. Whether the situation is a traumatic event, an addiction, pain, etc., you need to voice positive affirmations.

You tap the energy meridians and chant positive

affirmations to clear the "short circuit"—the
emotional block—from your body's bioenergy system.
This tapping procedure restores your body and
mind's balance, which is essential for optimal health
and healing physical disease.

An old saying is, "We should judge a tree by its
fruits." The outcomes of EFT can be quickly and
easily tested by learning the basics and initiating EFT
to work on eradicating any negative emotion. EFT
takes just 5 minutes to learn on the Internet, and
then you can put it to work and experience the results
of your own direct application.

6. Healing Touch (HT)

Healing Touch is an energy therapy that assists
mental, emotional, physical, and spiritual wellbeing.
It harnesses one's energy to support healing.

Like any holistic treatment, there are detractors;
however, Healing Touch is already easy to use. It is
used in long-term care facilities and hospitals, as well
as in hospices, private practices, and spas.

It was founded in 1989 as a continuing education

program for nurses, health care professionals, and massage therapists. It is taught in medical and nursing schools and universities.

WebMD delves into a study in which a group of women were being subjected to the threat of electric shock just by touching the hands of their husbands; they saw an immediate decline in their anxiety levels as their problems vanished.

There are a variety of symptoms that can be treated using Healing Touch, and a range of the issues that HT can be used to treat include, but are not limited to:

- Pain reduction
- Stress reduction
- Increased immunity
- A decrease in symptoms of anxiety
- In cancer care
- Surgery recovery

The American Holistic Nurses Association (AHNA) endorsed Healing Touch in 1997. Visit their website to find a practitioner in your area.

There are several energy therapies, in addition to "healing touch," that can give similar results, such as:

- Therapeutic Touch
- Reiki
- Qigong

Moreover, many of these techniques have been used for thousands of years by shamans and other Asian healers. These ancient healers brought us yoga and acupuncture. The principles of Healing Touch are based on the same philosophies.

What can you expect from a Healing Touch session?

1. Once you have found a reputable practitioner, they will start you off with a centering process. The idea behind this is to calm the mind and for the practitioner to focus entirely on the patient.
2. This is followed by the practitioner focusing their intention on the patient's highest good.
3. The practitioner will then begin by scanning your energy field; this will generally involve passing hands along the surface of your body, which allows them to note any imbalances in

the energy flow. These imbalances usually present as tingling, heat or cold, a feeling of pressure, or heaviness.

4. This allows the practitioner to select the correct technique for your needs. The practitioner will either make sweeping hand motions around the body or place their hands on the patient's body. This process should balance and realign the energy flow, which many issues, including pain, stress, or illness, could have disrupted.

5. Once your session is complete, the practitioner will assess the energy field again to ensure there has been a change in imbalances.

6. When your treatment has concluded, the practitioner will ground you to bring you back to an alert state. You will be invited to offer feedback and discuss what self-care techniques you can employ and whether that includes further sessions with the practitioner.

To prepare for a session, ensure that you wear comfortable clothing, as you stay fully clothed during the treatment, which can last up to an hour.

Attend prepared to discuss how you want to benefit from this treatment; your needs and expectations will dictate the method of approach your Healing Touch practitioner employs.

On your first visit, you must also complete a health questionnaire. A session usually costs $50 to $100, but a series of sessions will be cheaper individually.

7. Lomi Lomi

Lomi Lomi, also known as a "Loving Hands" massage, is so much more than a simple physical manipulation. Rooted in the richness of ancient Hawaii, this indigenous healing modality weds specific physical techniques with spiritual intent—a truly transformative journey for body and soul.

Origins and Significance

The Lomi Lomi massage has ancient roots in the Hawaiian Islands. It is indigenous and performed by native healing spirits known as Kahuna. This knowledge and art passed down through generations, serves physical healing and brings synchrony between an individual and his world. The name "Lomi Lomi" literally means "to knead" or "to rub," reflecting the massage's rhythmic, flowing movements that bring the waves of the ocean into your room.

Techniques and Philosophy

Unlike most massage techniques worldwide, including Swedish massage, Lomi Lomi entails long, flowing strokes with forearms, hands, and even elbows. This movement has been created to imitate natural elements for complete relaxation and emotional release. It is also usually done with the integration of traditional Hawaiian chants and prayers, which will give greater value to the therapeutic experience and even the connection to one's spiritual self.

Physical and Emotional Benefits

Other physical benefits of Lomi Lomi include the release of muscle tension, improved circulation, and increased flexibility. However, the results of this massage can also transcend to more than just the physical. In each stroke, one invokes good energy that enables the client to release negative emotions or trauma stored in the body, thus creating profound emotional healing.

Cultural Significance

Lomi Lomi is more than a massage; it's a mirror of respect for nature and the bonding of all three: mind, body, and spirit. It is one of the very ancient modalities that speak into the spirit of Aloha—taking one through feelings of harmony and balance within oneself and everything in nature.

Incorporating Lomi Lomi into Modern Practice

Today, Lomi Lomi massage finds its place in various renowned spas and wellness centers around the world. The treatment modality falls perfectly in place due to its holistic approach toward healing and the cultural aspects enriched in it. A practitioner should possess proper knowledge of the cultural background of Lomi Lomi along with training so that this age-old tradition is respected and, at the same time, effective therapy is provided using this.

Lomi Lomi massage offers a powerful alternative to conventional treatments, addressing both physical and emotional well-being. By embracing this ancient Lomi Lomi massage, we can see that it is a powerful alternative to other therapies because it deals with the physical and emotional sides. Based on the acceptance of this ancient Hawaiian healing tradition, one may be taken into the most profound state of relaxation, emotional release, and spiritual connection. On a personal level of healing or the path of professional training, Lomi Lomi provides a path toward holistic wellness and harmony.

8. Polarity Therapy

Polarity Therapy is a unique wellness practice used on various occasions when other typical means of balancing a person's energy flow may have failed. Many practitioners have multiple ways to check someone's polarity.

Polarity Therapy techniques used with energy medicine are used to restore a balance of the body's energy by applying touch, specific exercise, nutrition, eating habits, and mindful self-awareness. Polarity therapy is sometimes thought that someone is out of balance and that polarity therapy helps to bring them back in balance. Being in balance is also referred to as being in optimum health.

Who is credited for Polarity Therapy?

"The problem of healing involves the harmonious relationships of man's inner energies to those of the without. The struggle is as old as mankind."
~Dr. Randolph Stone

Randolph Stone (February 26, 1890 – December 9, 1981) founded polarity therapy, a complementary, holistic, spiritually-based energy healing technique that restores a person's polarity.

Polarity therapy is an alternative therapy that involves balancing the flow of your body's life energy to balance, increase, or maintain optimum health. Randolph Stone, a chiropractor and osteopath, developed this technology. Polarity therapy is also credited as polarity balancing and polarity energy balancing.

This type of therapy is influenced by the concepts of energy flow used in many ancient healing modalities. They state that polarity therapy may differ from those types of medicine, given the theory that positive and negative energy charges in the body's electromagnetic energy field govern the energy flow.

How do you reverse polarity?

Donna Eden's preferred method to reverse polarity is to use a stainless-steel spoon (one with enough strength (metal) in the steel to attract a magnet) and rub it over the bottom of the feet. This could correct polarity in the entire system. Consider rubbing the spoon over the body and in the energy field around the body.

Do our bodies have polarity?

The body does not have a north- and south-poled field; instead, it has a positive and negative magnetic field from which energy is produced, which is somewhat hard to comprehend, considering polarity as the north and south poles.

Polarity

The periodic concept of polarity, called electronegativity, is used to describe polarity. Electronegativity is the reaction of the atom's ability to attract electrons in a chemical bond. To determine the polarity of a bond, you must find the difference in

the electro-negatives of the atoms involved.
Therefore, you think of positive and negative fields as
having some connection.

Polarity is Determined.

The polarity of a bond is determined by a periodic
concept called electronegativity. Electronegativity is
an expression of an atom's tendency to attract
electrons in a chemical bond. To determine the
polarity of a bond, you must find the difference in the
electro-negatives of the atoms involved. Therefore,
you think of positive and negative fields as having
some connection.

Polarity Therapy How It Works?

Using polarity therapy, we can understand that
illness is caused by disruptions in the body's energy
flow, resulting in stress, lowering the immune system,
trauma, and many other diseases. Polarity therapy is
based on the concept that there are three types of
energy fields in our body:

- Long-line currents that run north to south
- Transverse currents that run east-west

- Spiral currents that start at the naval and expand outward

A therapist or anyone practicing polarity therapy can scan a person's body for energy blockages to locate or find them. The areas most concerning and affected are the shoulders, neck, and back, where symptoms include pain, discomfort, muscle spasms, and muscle tension.

Scanning blockages are identified using various techniques to clear the paths of energy fields, including spinal realignment and movement exercises. Practitioners sometimes incorporate other treatments like deep breathing, yoga, and hydrotherapy, which can be included in polarity therapy.

Uses for Polarity Therapy

In various alternative health practices, polarity therapy is said to help with the following health problems:

- Allergies
- Anxiety

- Arthritis
- Back pain
- Chronic fatigue syndrome
- Depression
- Headaches
- Irritable bowel syndrome
- Migraines
- Stress

Additionally, proponents of polarity therapy claim that it can also improve range of motion, increase energy, decrease pain, relieve stress, and reduce swelling. Some suggest that polarity therapy can stimulate our immune and fight off diseases. Many in the alternative health field feel that even cancer can be addressed in some cases as an imbalance in someone's body to be corrected with positive results.

Many different illnesses create stress or bring on disease due to the function of the immune system becoming weak and taking on an imbalance in the body. Therapies like Polarity Therapy can create an environment that creates a balance for the body, correcting these imbalances and restoring the immune system. The key to health is proper balance in all body areas—adequate sunlight, diet, exercise, nutrients, and positive mental views of our life.

Using Polarity Therapy for Stress

Many practitioners believe that polarity therapy helps reduce stress. Studies have found that those given polarity therapies had a greater reduction in stress levels, a greater sense of wellbeing, and improved health issues. In addition, polarity therapy groups showed much greater improvements in depression, pain, vitality, general health, and wellbeing.

Stress is known to cause many different types of sickness and disease. It attacks your body's weakest points. To fight off your imbalances, take steps to improve your wellbeing and surround yourself with a positive outlook.

Similarities between Polarity Therapy and Reiki?

Reiki and Polarity Therapy share similarities. Both work with the subtle energies of the body that underlie its functions. Both require hands-on positions, although Reiki can be performed at a distance.

Reiki involves what is known as an "attunement," an energetic initiation of the Reiki original masters to the current students.

Polarity Therapy uses techniques that connect the positive, neutral, and negatively charged universal life energy forces to enhance the life force within a problem or troubled area—determining whether mental, emotional, physical, or spiritual creates a free flow of the life force energy.

Both therapies are significantly enhanced by the practitioner's presence, purpose, intention, and passion.

9. Pranic Healing

Pranic Healing has been used to heal small groups for thousands of years. The goal is to get rid of any toxic energy in the energy body, including the field of energy surrounding the physical body. These impurities in the energy body might seep through to the physical and manifest themselves as diseases and illnesses.

What you eat affects your physical body.

Your energetic shield, which covers your body, also affects the health of your physical body. Both are important!

What Makes Up the Energy Body?

There have been scientific studies by Semyon Kirlian, the prominent Russian scientist behind the discovery of Kirlian photography. He photographed the aura of humans, animals, and plants using an ultrasensitive camera process. This specialized method, also known as electrography, showed a radiant, colorful field of energy around the physical body.

He called this electrical energy field the "aura" and described it as extending 4 to 5 inches from the skin's surface and capable of penetrating the physical body. Through his experiments, Kirlian discovered that the presence of disorders manifested themselves first in the energy body before appearing in the physical body.

He also noted that our thoughts, emotions, and moods directly affect our auras' vibrancy, radiance, and color. Our auras are a direct reflection of how we handle stress daily.

The Science Behind Pranic Healing

Prana is a Sanskrit word that means our "life force." If lucky and insightful, this life force keeps us alive and maintains good health.

One of the fundamental pranic healing principles is that our bodies can repair themselves from almost any ailment. We can step up this healing process by surrounding ourselves with positive life force energy and releasing the negative prana living within us (invading the body).

Pranic healing engages our energy field to release illnesses and sicknesses, from the mental to the emotional to the physical – anything has been proven possible!

You must also have positive thoughts to heal!

All pranic healers focus on wiping out the earmarks of disease.

You can be a professional, trained alternative medicine practitioner or do it yourself. It still works.

You can find an infected energy form in certain body parts, especially where you have pain. You can replace the ailing areas with clear, vitalized prana using the touch of the hands and following a specific "no-touch" approach. Hands-off still works well.

Pranic With No Physical touch

There is no physical contact since the practitioner works with the energy body rather than the physical body. The energy body may also be called the "aura," the energy surrounding our physical bodies. It absorbs life energy from everything around us, including the people, the sun, air, and wind, and distributes it to our physical human body.

Our muscles, glands, organs, cells, tissues, and other organs all receive the energy sent to us by our auras.

The pranic healers clean the energy body from any negativity or blockage spots before they come into the body, causing a problem.

Basic Principles Of Pranic Healing

Now that we understand pranic healing, we know it first brings balance and harmony to our energy body.

Next, our physical body receives that energy.

We need to appreciate the two fundamental principles of this alternative healing method.

1)   Law Of Self-Recovery

- The body can rejuvenate itself at an individual rate
- Your body will heal (from an injury, a cold, a cut, or a bruise, for example) in a week or two without resorting to going to a doctor for medication

2)   Law Of Life Energy Is All Around Us

- Prana ("vital principle") is the essence of life
- Whole body healing can be accomplished by integrating prana and strengthening its presence on the affected part

6 Steps To Pranic Healing

In Pranic Healing, there are 6 six steps to cleanse and transform the energy body.

In a few days, a group of practitioners maintains that the effects of these steps will show positive results, giving you an entire makeover of body and soul. There are, however, some steps whose effects will be felt immediately, such as pranic breathing. Still, together, these steps will add a recognition of ease and strength to your energy and physical body.

1. You will have help to clear your mind of all negative emotions and energy, including fears, anxieties, and phobias, as they block the flow of prana, which often leads to illness.

2. When achieving peaceful harmony requires that both energy and physical bodies be healthy.

It's fundamental to include physical exercise in the pranic healing ideology. The exercises target precisely the generation of energy. The exercises target the production of prana for the best benefits. They include but aren't limited to:

The Mental Physics Exercises and Tibetan Yogic Exercises.

We have simplified them while still ensuring they produce healthy, energized prana.

3. The pranic practitioner will manually manipulate your energy fields by scanning your body with their hands, allowing you to feel for any imbalance in your aura. Then, using specific sweeping motions, you can cleanse away the unclean parts of your aura.

Finally, use your hands again, draw in positive energy, and disburse it into your prana (aura) lacking areas to revive its energy field.

4. Just as the hygiene of your physical body is essential, so is the hygiene of your energy body. Regulating your emotions, following specific dietary recommendations, and many other ways are available to keep your energy body cleansed and purified.

5. We can only talk about alternative medicine by discussing meditation. To feel the maximum effects of pranic healing, there are numerous meditation techniques, but the two basic kinds are:

a. Mindfulness meditation: this method helps to slow down a person's flow of thoughts and facilitates the flow of cleansing energy

b. Meditation on Twin Hearts: this technique draws in vast amounts of healing prana by focusing on peace, kindness, and love

6. Breathing. We all know how to breathe as a biological process: in with the oxygen, out with the carbon dioxide. However, nearly every one of us is unaware of another fundamental aspect of our breathing process: our life force. The sad truth is that not many even know how to breathe right.

Breathing appropriately is the first step to increasing your energy levels. As we age, we allow stress and tension to constrain how we naturally breathe. We constrict our muscles, and they cannot expand and contract to their full span of movement. In a time of stress, we take deep breaths because we innately understand that this is how to loosen the diaphragm, thus allowing it to take in the maximum amount of oxygen.

However, there's another reason why breathing deeply calms us besides the physiological one; when muscles are relaxed, and breathing is rhythmic and slow, our bodies' paths of energy (chakras) become synchronized, resulting in the equilibrium of a sense of calmness and energy while at the same time experiencing tranquility and alertness.

Proper breathing techniques have great physiological benefits, such as:

- o Increase lung capacity
- o Provide a more proficient exchange of oxygen
- o Augment stamina levels
- o Decrease tension in muscles

- o Reduce anxiety
- o Enhance cardiovascular functions
- o Boost the immune system

Also, there are several prana benefits:

- More able to release negative energy that is trapped in the body
- A more purified energy body
- Aura rays become healthier and more vibrant
- Better ability to take in more significant amounts of positive prana

Pranic Healing Can Help Relieve Physical ailments:

- Headaches/ migraines
- Toothaches
- Coughs
- Stomach aches
- Muscle pains and sprains
- Cold/fever
- Back pain
- Hypertension
- Heart problems
- Arthritis

- Mental and emotional illnesses:
- Stress/anxiety
- Depression
- Phobias
- Addictions
- Relationship/financial issues

Your immune system will boost, and you will radiate energy.

It's essential to remember that pranic healing requires no physical touch to achieve its purpose. It deeply respects all philosophies and religions and is not associated with mystical or superstitious applications. Its fundamental intention is to complement traditional medicine, not to take its place in any way. It is also a perfect accompaniment to other alternative healing methods.

10. Quantum Touch®

Quantum touch can be a powerful energy healing technique that works with Universal Life Force Energy, similar to Reiki and Healing Touch. It helps the body reduce pain and promote optimal wellness.

Quantum touch is the use of natural healing energy to create optimal wellness. Energy healing is an alternative holistic practice that uses universal life force energy to locate and remove energy blocks and help stimulate the body's ability to heal.

Life Force Energy is from the universal source. It is also called the Universal Life Force. It can also be called 'chi' in Chinese and 'prana' in Sanskrit, is the flow of energy that sustains all living creatures. Some of us have more ability to sense its presence than others. It is all around us and a part of everything.

Can Quantum-Touch Energy Healing Work?

Healing with energy is a fascinating and natural process that is misunderstood.

 Although it may be hard to believe that we can heal other people through all types of energy healing, self-healing is possible! It is important to realize that all healing is self-healing and that all energy comes from the Source.

The human body has an extraordinary intelligence

and ability to heal itself using the God-given flow of energy.

 If the body has the right nutritional, energetic, emotional, and spiritual environments, its natural state is perfect health.

Are you a healer? My favorite definition of a healer is someone who was sick and got well; a great healer is someone who was extremely ill himself and got well quickly.

What is self-healing? Although all healing is self-healing, energy healing can assist other people in healing with their natural healing process. It involves teaching others to project and use or give a sense of energy sources.

What energies do Quantum-Touch and other energy healers use?

Quantum-Touch can include the basics of energy healing like Reiki, Pranic Healing, therapeutic touch, Healing Touch, etc., Using Universal life-force energy (known as prana in Sanskrit) and (chi in Chinese) to facilitate and promote healing.

The Quantum-Touch methods teach us to be in touch with ourselves, focus, and use our energy to amplify life force energy by using and combining various breathing and body awareness exercises.

Life-force energy is a necessary tool for healing; this is the principle of resonance and entrainment. In physics, as in nature, entrainment theory is the process where two vibrating objects at different speeds start to vibrate at the same rate. Then, the vibrational energy is transferred between the two objects, between the two people, or between humans and animals. Entrainment shows up in nature, chemistry, neurology, biology, medicine, things that vibrate, and more. For example, notice the clocks in your house are in sync, musical instruments will resonate together, crickets will chirp in unison, and fireflies will flash simultaneously.

We can use quantum touch techniques to create a powerful universal life force energy healing frequency. Suppose we use this frequency field of high energy around an area of pain, stress, inflammation, or disease. In that case, the body can entrain to the higher frequency, thus amplifying the body's ability to heal itself. For example, your cat climbs onto your lap and starts purring just as you are experiencing some discomfort in your right thigh. Within a short time, the pain subsides.

Quantum-Touch provides universal life force healing energy for the practitioner and the person seeking healing. Like Reiki, the practitioner will benefit from the flow of this energy. Using the QT techniques, the practitioner can hold an extraordinarily high vibration with a little practice. This high vibration is a healing flow of higher Source energy, and it influences the client but also provides a stream of healing energy for the practitioner. Like Reiki, you will feel refreshed and not drained from doing healing work; the practitioner is not using their own strength and will most often feel emotionally uplifted as a result! For those of you who have had the pleasure of being in the presence of a small baby, your touch can say it all: both parent and child are receiving the healing energy at once.

How do you know you are a healer?

    1) You're sensitive.
    2) You like being alone.

3) You're intuitive.
4) You have a big heart.
5) You are aware of the energy.
6) You enjoy helping others.
7) The word "healing" opens you up to a feeling of love.

Does therapeutic touch mean any of the following?

An alternative medicine technique in which the practitioner passes their hands over the body of the person being treated, creating a sense of calm, inducing relaxation, reducing pain, and helping promote healing. An energy shift is usually noticed within a matter of days, if not immediately.

You Can Learn About Reiki, Healing Touch, and Healing Touch Massage

One of the energy-based healing modalities, healing touch therapy is gentle and nurturing and takes place with a hands-on approach without invasive procedures, medications, or equipment. The practitioner places their hands lightly on or just above the individual. Sometimes, the energy transfer does not require touching the person or animal.

Is Healing Touch the same as Reiki?

Healing Touch is much like therapeutic touch and does not require an attunement, like Reiki before you can practice it. It is a modality that was recreated and developed by Janet Mentgen, RN and was originally for those in the medical field. However, it is now available to all. She noticed that using your hands (Healing Touch) became a method of altering the body's energy system to influence the self-healing and healing of a client.

11. Reiki

There Are Many Benefits of Reiki

Reiki promotes harmony and balance. It is a practical, noninvasive energy healing modality that enhances the body's natural healing ability while energizing and promoting overall wellness. Reiki works directly on restoring mental, emotional, and physical stability. It is a Source of energy flow that works directly on problems and conditions instead of just masking or relieving symptoms.

When we talk about stability and balance, we mean mental and emotional strength, left and right brain, male and female, not labeling things as good or bad, positive or negative, etc. Keep neutral about stuff because, in reality, there is no good or bad. There are things you want more of in your life, such as health, wealth, happiness, and joy. Wherever you put most of your attention – there you are! You must choose where you put most of your attention rather than letting your life be created from random thoughts!

Creates Deep Physical Relaxation and Helps the Body Release Stress and Tension

Many people enjoy Reiki treatment because it allows them time to themselves, where they aren't 'doing' but just 'being.' We are said to Be Human Beings, not human doings!

Clients have reported feeling more relaxed, bright, peaceful, and lighter in themselves after the first Reiki treatment.

Reiki provides a more spacious area where you can be aware of what is happening inside your body and mind. You can learn to listen to your body connection and make wise decisions from this place. What do you need for your wellbeing? You will benefit from being more present in your body, which will help you have even more inner knowing and wisdom that we should all have! Relax; you can also have abundance in all areas of your life.

Benefits of energy healing

1. Your hands can flow Source Energy for healing!
2. Your Reiki practitioner is trained to flow an unlimited amount of this energy
3. As a client, you only have to allow this Source energy to do its magic
4. Reiki Helps You Let Go of Energy Blocks
5. It promotes a natural balance between mind, body, and spirit.

Regular Reiki treatments can bring about a more peaceful, calmer state of being. After a Reiki session, a person can better cope with everyday stress. This mental/emotional balance also enhances learning, memory, mental clarity, and healing sickness.

Benefits of energy healing

Reiki can heal spiritual, mental, and emotional wounds, and it can help alleviate mood swings, fear, frustration, and even anger. Reiki can also strengthen and improve your personal relationships.

Reiki enhances your capability to love.

It can help you stop judging, open up to the people around you, and improve your relationships.

Reiki is high energy, causes the body to cleanse itself of toxins, and supports a healthier immune system.

High energy flow means you have a high flow of Life Force Energy that's necessary for healing!

People spend so much time in the stress-reactive fight/flight phase that it becomes our standard way of life, and our bodies may forget how to return to peace and balance. Disease is looking for people with stress and a low Life Force energy flow.

Reiki energy treatments remind our bodies to shift into the relaxed parasympathetic nervous system self-healing mode.

The parasympathetic nervous system is one of three divisions of the autonomic nerve system, and it helps to stop calling the body's nerve system nervous.

Nervous is a negative word. The way we talk about our bodies becomes its law.

It is also called the rest and digest system. When you are in the rest/digest body mode, you don't have to stop being active and productive or do nothing.

The parasympathetic system conserves your body's energy. It slows down the heart rate and increases intestinal and gland activity.

How to slow down even more?

1. Breathe Deeply with focused attention.
2. Specific breathing exercises may also be used to calm the nervous system.

It allows you to sleep better and digest better, essential to maintaining health and vitality. The more you are in this loving space, the more you can be active and productive without being anxious, stressed, exhausted, or burnt out.

Reiki Clears the Mind and Improves Focus as You

Feel Grounded & Centered

Healing energy comes out of your hands

Most people are not grounded, and they spend too much time worrying. Worry is simply a supercharged prayer for things you don't want. You can choose how you spend your time and where you focus your attention! Reiki will support you in staying centered in your heart and being in the present moment rather than getting caught up in shame, blame, regrets about past situations, or having stress and anxieties about the future. It can strengthen your ability to accept and work with how events unfold, even when they don't follow your desires or timetable.

Where there is Vibrational Harmony within yourself, you begin to react to situations, people, and yourself in a supportive way rather than acting out of habit and fear.

A Reiki Healing Session Accelerates the Body's Self-healing Ability, helping you return to your natural state of health and wellbeing.

Reiki healing quickly returns you to your natural state or at least gets your body moving in the right direction. Reiki is Source Energy in Motion!

Reiki is considered an energy medicine.

When we breathe better, our minds naturally settle. Science supports that. That means your breathing, heart rate, and blood pressure improve. Breathing deeper is one of the first things to happen during a self-practice or treatment received from someone else.

As respiration deepens, your body moves into the parasympathetic nerve system (PNS) dominance, i.e., the rest/digest phase. Your body was made to heal and rejuvenate in this phase rather than the more commonly experienced fight/flight phase.

Reiki Aids in A More Peaceful Sleep

The first outcome of a Reiki energy session is healing and relaxation. Often, clients experience deep relaxation and sometimes fall asleep during the session. When we're relaxed, we think more clearly, we sleep better, our bodies heal better, and we relate to each other more genuinely.

Reiki Helps Relieve Pain and Supports the Healing of Your Physical Body

If you only look at Reiki pictures, a Reiki treatment might appear merely a sequence of hand placements. However, Reiki energy comes directly from a higher Source and works to restore balance to you on the deepest possible levels. This stream of energy encourages your body to improve its vital functions (improving the physical body, breathing, digesting, and sleeping) so that your bodily systems function optimally.

On the physical level, Reiki helps to relieve pain from joints, migraine, arthritis, and sciatica ~ to name a few. It also helps with symptoms of depression, asthma, menopausal symptoms, chronic fatigue, and insomnia.

Reiki Helps Your Spiritual Growth and Emotional Cleansing

You do not need to be into spirituality to enjoy the benefits of Reiki. Many people receive Reiki energy treatments to support themselves through their self-healing journey of the body, mind, and spirit. Do you desire spiritual growth and personal development? Incidentally, the word spiritual is an internal mind quality and has nothing to do with religion; it is a direct connection to the supreme source.

Reiki energy addresses the whole person rather than targeting individual symptoms. This energy treatment can create profound, often subtle shifts from deep within your entire being.

What does spiritual growth look like?

Do you come from the heart (the feeling part of yourself), or do you come from the head (the thinking manipulating part of self)? Inner guidance about what to do in difficult situations can easily come from your heart. Or it may inspire a change in attitude or belief about your life direction. Suddenly, you see your stressful condition from a fresh perspective and can deal with it more positively. Opening your inner guidance system might direct you to the right action needed. This decision is guided by your connection to the God within, the Source of all, through your intuition.

Reiki Compliments Medical Treatment & All Other Therapies

A Reiki healing session is a beautiful complement to conventional medicine. It helps relax patients on the levels of the mind and physical body, accelerating the healing process. People sleep much better and are calmer following Reiki treatments.

The Reiki practitioner can give Reiki without touching the body in cases where patients do not want to be touched or have burns or significant injuries. The beauty of Reiki is that it is gentle and applied in a very peaceful manner.

Reiki is safe to use if you have medical conditions such as diabetes, epilepsy, or heart conditions. It is beneficial to receive Reiki treatments if you are undergoing chemotherapy for cancer.

A pregnant woman can have Reiki treatments to support her through all stages of the pregnancy.

Reiki is one of the few healing modalities you can use on yourself. After an attunement from a Reiki Master, your energy healing flow is increased forever!

Reiki is for everyone!

You Can Learn Reiki Yourself or Go to A Reiki Practitioner!

Many clients will become Reiki practitioners by attending my free Reiki Level 1 course at the Reiki Ranch to boost their daily energy levels. Some want to delve deeper into their spiritual and personal development. Some are drawn to Reiki to support their physical healing. Most have experienced the benefits of Reiki and wish to regularly be able to help themselves and others in the same way. Visit www.reikiranch.com for more information.

12. Laser Reiki

You Could Try an Energy Pain Release Treatment

Laser Reiki (LR) is the same loving energy as traditional Reiki, but it comes into your body at a higher frequency, increasing the natural healing energy your body typically attracts.

Experience a session or Learn Instant Pain Relief at the Reiki Ranch. This energy healing method is miles ahead of other modalities, very quick, and easy to do. Learn Laser Reiki, a simple way to identify the root cause of any ache or pain in the body, mind, or soul. Learn how to remove it at the root cause (the beginning of the problem). LR instantly removes pain and stuck energy.

A big difference with Laser Reiki is that the healing energy is applied to the energy body – a subtle body - before being toned down into the third dimension of physicality. It has been proven to be at least 10 times faster and more complete than all other types of energy healing modalities.

6th Dimensional Energy Is Used to Heal

When the practitioners used LR, the healing energy from Source entered the client at a 6th-dimensional level, which can be even higher depending on the practitioner's experience. It requires a precise spot for its application to the client's energy field.

Do you have any ongoing aches or pains? These energy-healing methods are excellent for relieving chronic pain because they release the root cause of that particular pain. Once the foundation of that pain system is removed, the pain itself usually follows and goes away.

Laser Reiki is Instant Pain Relief!

These methods will remove ongoing energy blockages causing chronic pain in the physical body from a traumatic experience, no matter when that root cause took place.

Whether the Cause of:

- The pain is in the present life
- In a past life
- From other lifetimes

- Or caused by dark energy from other dimensions and other realities.

Once the energy blockages are released with Laser Reiki's simple clearing methods, your health frequency will rise to a higher number, and the pain will instantly go away.

The LR energy flows out the fingertips like a laser beam — hence the name.

Laser Reiki clears the physical body and heals the energy body – the 6th level. (Laser Reiki is using energy to energy.) It is the most efficient use of Reiki and is at least 10 times stronger than traditional Reiki or any other energy healing method. With the energy body corrected for energy blockages, the flow of energy and the matrix of a perfect energy flow are restored. The new matrix will tell the physical body what to do – as above, so below! Instant healings occur in this manner.

This beam of energy is applied to the meridian of the central "nerve" system (not the nervous system— because we don't want to encourage nervousness in any of our body's systems). In other words, it is applied to a person's vertical midline. Laser Reiki is not used for the area of the pain. It will, many times, instantly remove the pain from the body. Those who feel the energy flow always experience an uplifting, happy feeling.

After an attunement to Laser Reiki, practitioners can flow at least 6th-dimensional healing energy and higher. This high flow of Source energy is one of LR's secrets.

You learn to find the root cause of the disease.

It is usually an unresolved emotional issue called an energy blockage. Energy blockages can be found at the mental, emotional, psychological, spiritual, psychic, genetic, or other levels, including the past, present, future, parallel, and other dimensional lives. They could bleed over from another "you" from your soul group or any lifetime where you had some negative experience.

The subconscious mind is used in LR and Cosmic Energetic Healing to find the exact location of energy blockages. It keeps all our aches and pains in the correct location until released. The subconscious mind is very powerful and has a wealth of information about your body—past, present, and future. It operates at all levels of energy and consciousness.

Laser Reiki practitioners constantly clear their energy blockages to be a clear and pure channel for the higher levels of this healing energy. It would be best if you cleared yourself first to be a good channel (pipe) for the higher source energy for your client.

It may take 1 to 3 sessions to heal asthma symptoms with Laser Reiki and release the root cause of the underlying emotional problem. In only one session, the client will notice a measurable improvement in the illness. Compare that to 30 to 40 treatments over 6 months using traditional energy healing Reiki or other methods to achieve the same results. MDs who only treat the symptoms may never clear the root cause of any disease.

LR Teaches You How to:

- Use Laser Reiki – a concentrated energy beam from the 6th dimension and above that flows out the fingertips.

- Discover the root cause of dis-ease and imbalances (what emotion or trauma started it in the first place.)
- An energy-to-energy process for removing pain, trauma, stress, anxiety, fear, etc. — instantly in most cases.
- Clear imbalances and/or dis-eases years before they become apparent.
- How to determine the amount of energy blockages in a person or situation.
- Clear hidden beliefs and hidden fears in Moments.
- Do remote energy treatments using only the person's name and location.
- Calculate and clear the reasons that are holding you back from success in all areas of your life.
- Heal yourself, your friends, your family, pets, and plants with Source energy.

One of our accomplished LR masters, Charles Miller, has pondered how deep Laser Reiki has gone since his training. Charles figured out what we are accessing, and I'll let him explain how deep this healing modality goes.

Reiki Is Energy In Motion

Reiki is one of the names given to energy in motion.

Traditionally, the name Reiki is associated with moving energy supporting the art of healing.

After working with this traditional practice for a while, I began to understand the hidden fundamentals of Reiki.

To me, Reiki is the fundamental energy emitted by creation itself. This energy makes up all things in all dimensions of existence.

By all things, I mean both dynamic energy, that substance which is in motion as in the life force of all living things, all-natural elements or combinations of elements arranged by creation, and static energy, fixed energy created by conscious rearranging natural energies.

A tree, a toad, a rabbit, a man – all are dynamic energy, as are water, rocks, rubies, a Thought.

All of this is from the Reiki energy arranged in nature

by the Reiki itself.

Steel, a wooden chair, and a car in all its parts are static energy, as are books or computers.

Dynamic energies organized in specific patterns are what mankind understands as life or natural elements.

When humanity alters, by intentional effort, adding to or deleting from these elements while reorganizing them into something useful, the original energies still exist, merely in a rearranged order resulting in static energy.

So, what is this ability to recognize natural elements and then reorganize them into something useful? The original energies still exist and have been rearranged, resulting in static energy. From where does this ability originate?

Consciousness!

So, what is consciousness?

Consciousness is energy moved in a specific manner.

So, the ultimate question is, where did all this energy, consciousness, and organized energy that makes up everything come from?

The following statement provides an adequate and competent answer.

The beginning of all things in this dimension of existence comes from the first thought.

Know Your Self

These three words explain the creation, and they all express forms of creation's energies in all places from the beginning. There are no limits on the expression of energy.

These three words invite infinite expressions of energy in motion.

1. Know
2. Your
3. Self

Once I engaged to Know My Self the recognition that

I was created by something larger than myself became clear.

The more I engaged to Know My Self, the more I recognized that if all creation is made up of the same stuff, all the things I am included, we all have common ground.

Once recognized, the common ground allowed me to understand that a shared source meant a common language, pure energy.

Laser Reiki is the tool for recognizing and working with, understanding, and participating in the dialogs of that language.

Accepting the gift of the language taught in this school and open dialogue from creation as a choice to engage allows me to know myself intimately and participate in the Neutral Flow of Creation's Energies. THE SOURCE!

The Ultimate Gift from Creation is the Choice!

Roi and Taylore developed and tested the Laser Reiki into a direct application, much like a phone app, available to anyone seeking to know themselves and make sense of this wild experience we call life (on Earth).

By Charles Miller

13. Restorative Touch™

Restorative Touch™ seeks to support health, healing, and spiritual evolution. It was developed from our increasing quest for past, present, and future modalities.

What is Restorative Touch™?

Restorative Touch™ is a unique method of energy work created and developed by the Vibrational Health Institute. As Certified Restorative Touch™ Practitioners, they work to restore vitality and a sense of harmony in your client by aligning their energy fields to their maximum potential.

Upon receiving Restorative Touch™, in addition to a unique increase of radiance, clients often report a deep sense of wellbeing and feeling at home with themselves. Clarity, self-knowledge, awareness of the deeper self, and a sense of a way to pursue innovative endeavors or resolve existence's challenges have been shown to improve from just one Restorative Touch™ session.

Although Restorative Touch™ isn't always a choice to scientific care, reducing or resolving bodily, mental, and/or emotional pain is not unusual upon receiving Restorative Touch™ strength work.

While all sorts of energy healing share a few commonalities, they have a few specific distinctions.

While most energy recovery channels use external power, they work with the lively resonance of the recipient's maximum potential, calibrating and aligning their body and subject to that maximum potential.

Practitioners work mainly with their hands in the clients' energy fields, working to balance and align the energy fields and open up their healing potentials.

As part of helping humans align their maximum potential with their core essence, it also allows recipients to fully express their center essence in the physical world, cultivating the recipient's private vitality and contributing to a lifestyle that fulfills their deepest, purest longings while uniquely serving the world.

Health and healing are regarded through this lens. Practitioners may work with the energy fields and chakras, as well as different components of the active anatomy, clearing and balancing as many other types of power work do, but additionally calibrating to the power signature of the individual's highest potential.

Thus, the work is highly specialized to the individual and supportive of the recipient's uniqueness.

Many have been using these techniques after many years of reviewing different techniques that are proven to work on balancing the body's energy centers. Some ancient cultures have incorporated many of the methods of Restorative Touch that were discovered on their own by trial and error working with people. For those wishing to extend their tools of healing modalities, there are places you can go for certification.

Developed by Daphne Michaels, founder and

president of the Daphne Michaels Institute, it is based on a version of reality and consciousness known as the Vibrational Paradigm. The Vibrational Paradigm is a work frame created from Michaels' incorporated view of psychology, philosophy, cutting-edge physics, and historical knowledge traditions. Like most types of energy healing, the Vibrational Paradigm views the universe and its entirety as energy.

Certified practitioners go through at least four years of schooling. The four-year training fosters growing private active radiance and a cultured mild body (developing a cultured energetic presence), increasing consciousness, living consciously, studying the use of intention, and embodying one's complete potential. Practitioners are licensed, held to high ethical standards, and must undergo continuing education. Most practitioners are within the Pacific Northwest location of the US, close to the Tacoma-based totally Daphne Michaels Institute. Many combine RT with other professions.

The Daphne Michaels Institute (formerly the Vibrational Health Institute) is a Washington State-licensed vocational school committed to human development.

Since many are unfamiliar with these techniques, you can search for a practitioner who can use them on your body to help you locate and balance your energy flow and regain a more vibrant, healthy life. These techniques allow your body to take over and rejuvenate your energy-healing powers.

14. Shamanic Healing

Every night, when we go to sleep, we go on a 'shamanic journey.' When we dream, our soul leaves our body to explore other worlds as an 'unconscious' journey into the spirit world. We also leave our bodies when we experience trauma, as our soul tries to protect itself. Our souls leave the body for several reasons, but few of us can leave the body at will; this is where shamanic training comes in.

Before being able to intentionally leave the body and embark on a 'shamanic journey,' many shamans will first have to go through a near-death experience, which, in a way, shows the shaman what it's like to leave the body and will make it less likely that they will be alarmed when the time comes to leave the body at will for shamanic healing.

The shaman must first enter a 'trance-like' state to induce a shamanic journey. Special music or drumming may mimic the Earth's frequency or 'heartbeat' and relax the mind. The shaman must also make an 'intention' for the journey, call on spirit guides, and ensure they are well-protected before entering another realm.

A shaman might go on a journey to perform shamanic healing, communicate with spirits, retrieve a soul, or meet with their spirit animal.

Three Levels

Journeying to the unseen' spirit world', you will discover that there are three levels or 'worlds':

The Lower World

The lower world is where our ancestors and spirit animals reside. This realm is deeply connected to nature and has an earthy feel. In shamanism, it is believed that all thoughts and ideas are stored, sorted, and processed in a metaphysical realm that shamans can access during their spiritual journeys. This realm is also referred to as the underworld, which shamans can enter through various means, such as a hole in a tree or by going into a pond.

The Middle World

The Middle World is very similar to our earthly plane. It's a multidimensional world filled with various thought forms, extrasensory perceptions, and hidden energies. If a shaman is looking to find a cure for a shamanic healing ceremony, they would enter the Middle World for the answer to what ails the sufferer. This world is considered challenging to navigate due to its many layers.

The Upper World

The upper world is the spitting image of heaven, where spirit guides, angels, and cosmic beings reside. Their guidance is normally more 'philosophical' and less practical than guides from the lower world. This realm is often entered when the shaman needs to channel 'divine guidance' on healing a terminal illness during a shamanic healing session.

How Shamanic Healing Works

When it comes to shamanic healing, the shaman essentially works in tandem with spirits, often called 'helper spirits,' in the spiritual realms. They will 'summon' these spirits to repair a soul, who may experience natural, physical healing in the earthly realm. To contact these spirits, the shaman must journey by entering a trance state. The more practice and training a shaman has, the easier it will be for them to enter this powerful state.

The shaman might ask their helper spirits to invoke shamanic healing by pulling 'power' from the sufferer's oversoul and retrieving lost spirit guides and animals.

People who have been through a life-altering trauma, whether mental or physical, may have lost a part of their soul or damaged their 'spiritual force field,' making them vulnerable to illness, bad luck, and depression. These are the kinds of people who would most benefit from a shamanic healing session. A shaman will go into the spirit world and heal their soul through their own efforts or by talking to spirit guides/animals.

Is Shamanic Healing Right For Me?

If you feel a little 'lost' in life, have gone through a significant trauma, or are looking for some clarity on what to do about a problematic situation, a shamanic healing session could be hugely beneficial. A shaman will connect you and your guides in the other realms and ensure your soul is protected throughout the process. Some physical sensations may be felt, but it's all in the interest of healing your soul.

Some people opt to learn shamanic healing for themselves rather than consult a shaman. The truth is, anyone can take a shamanic healing journey. It's all a matter of training yourself to get into the right state and knowing what to do once you are in other worlds. Thousands of people can 'astral project 'into the spirit world, but it takes a shaman to go into these worlds with intention and knowledge of how to heal.

Honoring the world of form and spirit and surrendering to endless death and rebirth is the Source of all healing—the shaman's power.

15. Shiatsu

In Japanese, Shiatsu means "finger pressure." For shiatsu massage, the therapist uses varied, rhythmic pressure on certain precise points of the body. These points are called acupressure points, and they are believed to be important for the flow of the body's vital energy, called chi. Proponents say shiatsu massage can help relieve blockages at these acupressure points.

Shiatsu is a form of therapeutic bodywork that originated in Japan. The techniques commonly used are kneading, pressing, soothing, tapping, and stretching techniques. Massage without oils through light, comfortable clothing.

Shiatsu means "finger pressure." It is one of three systems that developed in Japan in the early 1900s because of a merging of traditional therapies, including acupuncture and massage. Shiatsu evolved from conventional Japanese manual therapies with modern Western medical knowledge.

How can Shiatsu advantage your health and wellbeing?

Shiatsu is a noninvasive healing remedy that reduces pressure and promotes wellbeing. It also treats various internal, emotional, and musculoskeletal conditions.

- Lessons muscle stiffness
- Stimulates the Skin
- Balance the digestive system
- Open energy pathways
- Body Life Force energy system

Shiatsu is used to treat a wide range of chronic conditions:

- Headaches
- PMS
- Digestive disorders
- Fatigue
- Insomnia
- Fibromyalgia
- Stress
- Anxiety
- Musculoskeletal pain
- Low back

- Neck
- Joint pain

Depending on the session's intention, the effects can be stimulating, invigorating, calming, and soothing.

You need to specify the amount of comfortable pressure for your body type. Some people are more sensitive than others. I prefer a relatively soft touch in massage. The effects of the massage may take up to a day to feel. Some people feel sore after a massage of this type.

Principles of Shiatsu?

One fundamental Chinese/Japanese medicine concept is Qi (pronounced "chee"), the vital life force energy in our body that underlies all your energetic functioning.

Qi flows in your pathways, called meridians. The Shiatsu therapist accesses the Qi through exact energy points along the meridians, called Vital Points. Health and wellbeing are present when there is abundant Qi in our meridians, and the flow is unobstructed and balanced. Symptoms can arise

when the Qi becomes out of balance or deficient, or
the flow is obstructed.

Some of the symptoms and minor signs emerge, such
as:

- Regular colds
- Flu's
- Weekly or daily headaches
- Body aches
- Muscular pain
- Digestive difficulties.

These can be indications of an imbalance of Qi.
Shiatsu can help by stimulating and harmonizing the
flow of Qi throughout the body.

Shiatsu therapists are trained to recognize patterns of
disharmony in the body, often before physical signs
appear. Many simple yet subtle changes may indicate
an imbalance that, left alone, may progress to a point
where symptoms can occur. In most cases, balance
can be restored through proper assessment and
regular Shiatsu sessions. Shiatsu practitioners may
also offer lifestyle, diet, and exercise activity

recommendations.

Shiatsu as a therapeutic form of acupressure.

Shiatsu is a therapeutic form of acupuncture, muscle meridian stretching, and corrective exercising that originated in Japan. Shiatsu includes applying stress and pressure to the body using a person's thumbs, palms, elbows, knees, and feet. It is based on the standards of traditional Chinese medicine, which states that energy moves through channels in the body called meridians. Shiatsu practitioners aim to restore the stability of the energy through meridians correcting the energy flow, instilling means for the body to repair itself, and obtain optimum health and wellbeing.

Shiatsu is a dynamic method for body energy balancing, wherein the therapist interacts with the receiver to repair balance in the body's energic system. Imbalance, that is, too little or an excessive amount of chi, can manifest in diverse ailments, depending on which meridians are affected.

Like other natural therapies, Shiatsu is based on the idea that the body is a self-recovery organism and that the practitioner's function is to aid and support that naturally occurring process. Shiatsu can help a person with self-improvement and self-healing, balancing the underlying causes of a circumstance and addressing physical and mental functions, promoting health, and strengthening the body's recuperation abilities.

Although Shiatsu translates from the Japanese as' finger strain,' the thumbs, palms, elbows, knees, and feet apply pressure to diverse body parts. The pressure can be mild or firm, depending on the circumstance being treated.

Treatment may include flowing stretches and mild rotations of the limbs and joints, easy structural alignments, and muscle release techniques. On a physical degree, this stimulates flow and the flow of lymphatic fluid. It also works on the autonomic nervous system, releases toxins and deep-seated tension from the muscles, and can boost the hormonal system. On a subtler stage, Shiatsu allows the receiver to relax deeply, stimulating the body's inherent capability for self-healing and regeneration.

The man or woman receiving Shiatsu is dressed in

light clothing or covered by a sheet; bodywork usually occurs on a flat surface. Massage chairs that can be programmed are said to produce a shiatsu massage. Most people prefer personal touch massage over an electronic device.

Shiatsu's effectiveness in maintaining balance can be supported by recommendations concerning diet, yoga, meditation, and exercise as part of an overall remedy regime.

As with any body massage or energy work performed, it is wise to consider your conditions and consult a medical professional about any pre-existing conditions before any adjustments. It is always better to be safe than end up with additional complications.

Shiatsu massage is not for everyone. If you are unfamiliar with the type of massage, you should always start on the mild side and specify to the person giving the massage the amount of pressure to apply.

Note that your body has definite energy points; some call them chakras, others call them acupressure points, meridians, and Qi; they all come from the same Life Force Energy Source Points. When these are out of balance in anyone's body due to natural causes, diet, stress, or excess physical activity, these can be easily adjusted with recommendations referring to the natural cause. Other circumstances take time to recognize and correct. For example, exposure to toxic chemicals, accidents that cause damage to muscles, bones, and skin, and unnatural injury may need to be more examined to produce the best treatment and ways to move forward. First, we must locate the source of the issue or pain and proceed cautiously regarding the treatment. All of these natural and unnatural issues tend to block our energy flow, and our goal is to have our Qi function to its maximum at all times, creating a very exceptional sense of wellbeing as an energetic, fulfilled individual.

Conclusion

In conclusion, the journey of Lyme disease is profoundly personal, and each person's experience may vary in its symptoms, duration, and impact. Chronic Lyme disease, in particular, has proven to be an elusive and challenging condition, with traditional medicine often offering limited relief through symptom management rather than a cure.

Through our personal experiences and the insights shared in this book, we've aimed to provide a comprehensive look at the alternative therapies that have brought relief to many—including those treatments that exist beyond the conventional approach.

The need for a broader exploration of treatments stems not only from the experiences of those living with Lyme disease but also from the medical professionals who, after trying standard treatments, have found comfort and healing in alternative methods. While there are risks associated with exploring these lesser-known approaches, the overwhelming anecdotal evidence from our conferences and individual journeys suggests that these therapies hold promise.

Medical professionals and Lyme sufferers alike must navigate the field of alternative treatments with an open mind but grounded caution. We recognize the medical community's complex legal and professional barriers regarding recommending or acknowledging these therapies. Still, increasing awareness can lead to a more compassionate and holistic understanding of Lyme disease care.

As you close this book, we encourage you to take the knowledge shared here as a foundation for further exploration. Continue seeking information, speaking with alternative practitioners, and advocating for broader treatment options.

Chronic Lyme disease may be challenging to understand fully and even more difficult to treat, yet the persistence, adaptability, and courage of those living with Lyme are unmatched.

We hope this journey will empower and inspire you to seek holistic avenues of healing that resonate with your body and spirit.

May this be a step toward the relief, recovery, and quality of life you deserve.

Incidentally, the thing that worked for us in our quest to get rid of chronic Lyme disease was chlorine dioxide. Of course, we used Laser Reiki to take away the tendancy to contract a weird disease of any kind. That was over 12 years ago and nothing else has bothered us since.

Sending you healing love and light,

~Herb Roi Richards and Taylore Vance

You may contact us at Reiki Ranch dot com.

NOTES: